# Journey

*Experiences with Breast Cancer*

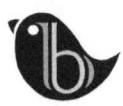

*This book has been a labour of love.*

*Many people have put countless hours into it, without renumeration.*

*Special thanks go to the authors.*

*Thank you for being brave enough to share your story and in doing so, helping others travel their own difficult journey.*

*To Christine and Sara,*
*who first inspired this book.*

Busybird Publishing
2/118 Para Road
Montmorency, Victoria
Australia 3094
www.busybird.com.au

First published by Busybird Publishing & Design 2012

Chief Editors: Blaise van Hecke and Les Zigomanis
Assistant Editors: Jodie Garth, Marieclaire Vandenberg, Laura Bovey
Poetry Editor: Krystle Herdy
Proofreaders: Lauren Grosvenor, Blaise van Hecke, Les Zigomanis
Cover Image: Kev Howlett
Layout and Design: Blaise van Hecke

Typeset in Palatino 11.5/18pt

National Library of Australia Cataloguing-in-Publication entry:

Title: Journey : experiences with breast cancer/chief editor, Les Zigomanis;
editing team, Marie-Claire Vandenberg [et al.]

ISBN 9780987153807 (pbk.)

Subjects: Anthologies. Cancer--Patients--Biography. Breast cancer patients'
writings.

Other Authors/Contributors: Various

Dewey Number: 614.5999449092

**DISCLAIMER:** The producers of this book, and the authors of the stories are not
medical professionals. It is not intended as a medical diagnostic tool but rather a
guide to help anyone facing breast cancer. Always seek medical advice and second
opinions where your health is concerned.

# Contents

# Foreword

On 8 August 2008, just before starting afternoon clinic, I listened to a message from my GP asking me to call him. Looking back, my body knew what that message was about. I still had an afternoon of clients to see, so I pushed it aside while I listened to other people's problems for the afternoon.

Later on that rainy Friday evening I left the private breast clinic alone, feeling like I wasn't in my own body. The words 'the lump is cancer, but we're not sure about the spots on your liver' didn't feel like they referred to me.

So began a journey. A journey that would impact on me, my husband, my children, my parents, my siblings and even my dog! It was a slog, but perhaps a journey that benefited us all in some way. We all got to know each other in new ways. Some had to take on new more challenging roles, some had to let go of outdated ways of doing things.

For all of us, it was life changing.

The stories in this book reflect different journeys through cancer. Many recount the story of their diagnosis; the moment by moment recounting of every test, every mood, the colour of the paint on the walls, the words uttered from oncologists' mouths. Every detail that stays with you forever. Almost as if that is the marker of life before cancer (BC) and life after cancer (AC). Breast cancer has almost become a rite of passage. For those who go on this journey, the cancer sufferers themselves or those around them, life is never the same.

My own journey led to me expanding my psychology practice to working with women with breast cancer. The themes in therapy are also represented in these stories: the trauma of diagnosis; the fear of recurrence; the new appreciation for life; navigating the medical system – for good and for bad; feeling angry, scared and alive; facing up to death; finding new meaning; examining relationships; sore arms; lymphodema. For the reader who is possibly undergoing their own journey, there is comfort in this. At some level, a normalising, that we are not alone in the suffering regardless of where our cancer might take us. In other people's stories we search for clues that might enhance our own survival.

Three years later, I am possibly the healthiest I have been in twenty years. At the time of diagnosis, a triple negative cancer with lymph node involvement gave me a seventy percent chance of being alive in five years. That was a scary figure to digest at the time. I think, it also gave me the impetus to change some things in my life. For me, the question was what can I control and what can't I? I could control diet, stress and exercise. Sticking to a healthy regime makes me feel empowered. I'm a bit sick of ongoing doctor's visits but don't yet want to let them go. Part of me says, *it won't come back* and the other says, *if it does, I will deal with it, just like I did the first time!*

Sara Van Hecke
Psychologist (Clinical)

# High Maintenance

*Jan Sutton*

I like to think of myself as low maintenance, but lately my life has changed.

This morning before school drop-off, I obediently cleanse and tone my face and apply some liquid make-up over the dark rings under my eyes, just like I've been shown to do. Next comes moisturiser, a light dusting of powder and a little blusher. There, don't I look better? Eyeliner is a regular for me, but I also apply some neutral eye-shadow. Then there's lip liner and a soft lipstick. Do I do this for myself, or to make others comfortable? I'm not sure. Either way, it does lift my mood, compensating for the fact that we now have even less time than usual to get to school.

'Come on, Mum, *you're* holding *me* up this morning,' says eight-year-old Carly.

Mid-morning, I notice the nail polish on top of the dresser near the door to the laundry, and I squat on the terracotta tiles and paint my nails with white hardener. Nobody can say I don't obey doctor's orders. *Tick!* No yellow, splitting nails for me.

All this effort, but I'm having a bad hair day. My part has widened, and there is a never-ending stream of hair strands on my shoulders. I choose a hat to disguise the thinning, and I go out.

\*\*\*

I catch a glimpse of myself in a shop window. It's a trendy hat, but I realise that beige is not really my colour, and underneath the hat, my face looks miserable.

\*\*\*

At home again, I scrutinise myself in the bathroom mirror. My scalp stings with the slightest pressure on my hair. It's inevitable, and I hate the waiting. I've made my decision. I hop in the shower and I massage and brush my hair. It's the longest shower I've had in a long while and I feel vaguely guilty. By the end of it, there is a massive pile of dark hair interlaced with grey, piled up on the white tiles in the corner of the shower recess. I may regret this; perhaps I should've hung onto it for a few more days.

I see myself in the mirror as the steam clears. I am bald, but for a wispy covering of hair, which makes me look old and sick. I'm not sick; the chemotherapy is prophylaxis. And I'm not old; just middle-aged. I'm not shocked either; I've been here before.

I get my wig out of its box. It's a few shades darker with auburn highlights. It's my first experience of a wig: high maintenance.

'Everyone will just think she's *finally* dyed her hair,' said a friend when I canvassed her about the option of a wig. Right, I get the message.

'I want you to wear a wig. I don't want you wearing a banner to school,' dictated Carly.

'It's a bandana, Carly, not a banner,' I corrected her, whilst thinking, yes, a bandana is a bit like a banner which screams, *I'm having chemotherapy!*

No bandanas, so, a wig it is. I don the thing. It's not too bad. Like I've had a dye job and got the hair straighteners onto it. A bit bouffy, though. Big hair is really not me. I try to brush it down, with little success.

\*\*\*

I go to school pick-up wondering if I can carry it off. I look sideways at all the mums to see if they are looking at me. Sure, it's a bit longer than my hair was yesterday. *Yeah, sometimes she cuts it long, sometimes she cuts it short, next time she'll cut it with a knife and fork,* is my silent quip to unspoken, imagined judgements. The hairdresser didn't have any appointments this afternoon to trim it for me. Do I look enviable? Do I look tarty? Or do I just look like I'm wearing a wig?

Carly's eyes are wide. She seems to get that it's a secret. She saw it at home, so she'll be right. She approaches me and pulls gently on both sides of my hair.

'Mum, I don't like it,' she tells me in a low voice.

'Don't pull it.'

'It looks funny.'

'Thanks.' Not the reception I was looking for. Ideally she wouldn't have even noticed. A big ask, I know.

\*\*\*

I'm relieved to be out on the footpath heading for the car. But she's not finished.

'Mum, why did you get that wig? It looks really stupid.' Louder now.

'Carly, I got this wig because you said you wanted me

to get a wig. I paid a lot of money for it.' I hate myself for laying the guilts on her.

'But, Mum, I meant,' she's saying slowly and loudly through clenched teeth, 'I meant for you to get one that didn't look STUPID! It looks stupid, stupid, stupid!' She's yelling at me now, with shadows of tantrums from days gone by. I start to giggle. Perhaps it's today's dose of nausea-preventing steroids, which allow me a sense of humour. After all, she has always been a drama queen, my daughter.

'Carly, if I wasn't laughing right now, I'd be crying.'

She doesn't let up. 'You have wasted your money, Mum. I hate it, hate it, it's so stupid!'

'I've got something for you at home,' I try to change the subject and succeed until we get back to the car.

\*\*\*

In the car, I figure it's safe to have a proper discussion. She's crying and the message is repetitive.

'Do you think it's stupid because it looks a bit bouffy?' I ask.

'Yes, it's really bouffy,' she declares. 'It's bouffy at the sides and bouffy at the back and it's bouffy where the fringe is.'

'Yes, it is a bit, isn't it? But lots of women go around with bouffy hair.'

'It looks really horrible.' At least the adjective has changed. 'Where are we going?'

'We're going to meet Aunty Marg at a café.'

'But, Mum,' she groans loudly, 'I'll be too embarrassed. I want to go home.' She's crying loudly, playing a different record. Tough love. As I drive through the slow-moving traffic, Carly bawls and yells discouragements all the way. Again I find myself giggling. Surely I don't look that bad?

***

'Hi, Carly, hi, Clare,' Marg is waiting at the 7-Eleven on the corner. Hugs and kisses all round. We walk to the café, Carly holding Marg's hand.

'What did you do today?' Marg asks me, as we sit down.

'I had a couple of appointments. And then I washed my hair off.'

Double take. 'Is that a wig? I didn't even notice. I just thought your hair was looking nice, that you'd had it straightened.'

'Did you hear that, Carly? Aunty Marg didn't even notice.'

Carly gives me a half smile from across the table.

'Can I tell Dad what you said about my wig?' I ask her when we're home again.

'Yes,' she reluctantly agrees. I relate part of Carly's reaction to Greg, and we both laugh. Carly frowns at me and pouts, and comes to sit on my lap.

'I don't like it when you laugh at me.'

'We're not laughing at you; it's just that we both got a shock. You were shocked because you wanted your old mummy back. And I was shocked because you didn't like my wig.'

'Yes, we were shocked.' She seems placated by this summary of events. But I am not so easily reassured; I definitely preferred my life when I was low maintenance.

# In Denial

*Jennifer Bryce*

I was waiting, waiting ... under the fifteen foot high architraves of a converted Victorian mansion. I pretended to read a magazine, having long ago abandoned the novel and the work I had brought. It had been a day of sitting on ill-assorted vinyl covered chairs that in no way matched the style and dignity just discernable in the massive nineteenth century rooms. I had been called back after my regular breast screen scan because something was 'not quite clear'. I progressed through each of the various stations in the breast screening centre without release; a more detailed scan, then an ultrasound, culminating now in the surgeon's waiting room.

And then his voice boomed down the marbled corridor: 'I need a social worker for the next ...'

The 'next' was me. So I knew before I went in that I would be told I had breast cancer. He needed a social worker to be there to cope with my expected despair. But I had sensed much earlier in the day that this would be my fate.

The social worker was young. I was fifty-three. Mine was not a textbook reaction and she was clearly at a loss. 'She's in denial,' I heard her tell the surgeon as I left the room at the end of the consultation.

My main memory of that consultation is the anger I felt at the patronising way I was treated by the social worker. I guess a psychologist would say that I projected my anger onto her. I don't remember everything I said, but I did say, 'Breast cancer is not the worst thing that has ever happened to me.'

And it isn't.

Twelve years earlier, my son had died at the age of sixteen months after spending his life in hospital. And just six weeks ago my husband had died. So many times I had wanted to be able to share their pain – to carry some of the burden of their illnesses myself. There was a sense of 'it's my turn now', even though I was in no way thinking of death. It was convenient that the surgery was to be performed a week before Christmas. I would be in hospital for the festive season – I could postpone a first Christmas without Graeme.

There was some disbelief, but not denial. I had not expected to get breast cancer. I wasn't close to anyone else who had had it. I had thought about the seeming brutality of total mastectomy compared to cutting out a 'lump'. But I had not really imagined myself in that situation. And now there was not much time to think about it.

The surgeon wanted to operate as soon as possible – I chose a lumpectomy. I pleaded to wait until after a garage sale I had organised for two weeks' time. So, the day after the garage sale, with a bag slung over my arm, feeding and walking of the dog organised, and wearing rather uncomfortable shoes, I walked down the bush track to the Woodend Station to catch the train to Melbourne for my operation.

In hospital I shared a room with a Greek woman who didn't speak English. We would mime our reactions to the meals that were brought in. I was worried that she was bored. Being enterprising I located the Occupational Therapy Library and borrowed some books in Greek – from the covers they looked as though they were adventure stories. But from her mouthing of the words, I think they were rather inappropriate. The same assistant surgeon visited both of us. One day this supposedly meek and compliant woman startled me by jumping out of bed after he had left and doing an excellent impersonation!

It took some days for us to be told the results of our surgery. One day we were told that the assistant surgeon would give us our pathology results around lunch time. In retrospect I am surprised by the level of anxiety I felt. After all – breast cancer is not the worst thing to have happened to me …

All morning I felt as though I was waiting in the wings to play a concerto; my stomach was churning and my heart pounding. When the assistant surgeon did come, the Greek woman's results were good and mine were relatively bad: seven out of eleven lymph nodes were cancerous and they had not 'cleared the margins' of my tumour, so I would need to have further surgery. I would be offered chemotherapy, radiotherapy and adjuvant therapy to prevent the return of cancer and to destroy any invasive cancer cells.

Looking at notes in my diary from that time, I see that I must have been concerned that the radiotherapy might affect my heart – it was my left breast. I opted for the most aggressive chemotherapy – my approach was take all that is offered. Imagine if the cancer returned; you would think, *If only I had taken the full treatment* … So the chemo and radiotherapy took up most of the following year.

I have a phobia of wigs. I think it goes back to a doll losing her hair when I was very young. So aggressive chemotherapy, with its side effect of hair loss, was a significant challenge for me. Nevertheless I opted for it, kidding myself that I would be in the 0.05 percent of the population who do not lose their hair. Of course, I was wrong. I remember sitting in a train carriage by an open window on a hot evening, aware that my hair was actually being blown away. So I massaged my scalp with lavender oil, used baby shampoo and did everything possible to retain my hair. I didn't lose all of it, although what remained was stiff and brittle – I'm sure a good brushing would have got rid of the lot. But I clung to it and avoided using a wig by covering my head with the many beautiful scarves that friends gave me. They desperately wanted to do something – my scarf collection was massive.

The other effects of chemotherapy were not nearly as bad as I had imagined. It felt a bit like the early stages of pregnancy, a slight queasiness settled by nibbling dry biscuits or sultanas. I was particularly touched by the generosity of the nursing staff who were aware that I was newly alone. The day after my first chemo session the head nurse phoned me at home to see if I was okay. I felt slightly guilty as I was eating a delicious lunch with a friend who had arrived with a bottle of wine – I hadn't expected to feel like drinking wine.

I was grimly determined that life would go on. In fact, I wanted to prove to the world that I could manage. This was a case of managing as a new widow as well as a person being treated for cancer. No way was I prepared to be a victim. With the executor, we were still negotiating Graeme's will. I was short of money, though I did have a secure job, which the bank manager didn't seem to appreciate. He suggested I sell the house, keeping the lower paddock on which I could place a 'mobile home'. Graeme owed money on his credit card, which the bank was prepared to write off. I was so incensed by the patronising attitude that I insisted on personally paying off the debt. I changed banks as soon as it was paid and I did not opt for a mobile home.

I desperately wanted to get on with a new life of independence. The breast cancer experience was a kind of bridge between the medical dependence, anger and profound regret of my son and Graeme's deaths and the busy life I lead now as a completely independent person. So while I was on chemotherapy I started a PhD, tentatively pushing open a door onto greater academic involvement and specialisation at work.

For me, the worst part of the breast cancer treatment was radiotherapy, maybe because it came after nine months of chemotherapy. Being locked alone in a room of smooth surfaces and humming machines was like being immersed in a 1950s science fiction story. I have never taken to science fiction. And it seemed crazy to submit to being burnt in the same spot day after day; like exposing bad sunburn to more sun.

After all this, the usual 'gold standard' adjuvant treatment would be the drug Tamoxifen. But my oncologist told me that I would be eligible to go on a drug trial – the ATAC trial of Anastrozole, Tamoxifen alone or in combination. The trial drug, Anastrozole had been successfully used for treatment of more advanced breast cancer. It was a Phase III trial, which indicated that Anastrozole was known to be safe for human consumption. It had been used with people who had more advanced breast cancer. This trial was to see whether Anastrozole was a better treatment than Tamoxifen for patients with what is termed 'early breast cancer'.

A main difference between Anastrozole and Tamoxifen is that Anastrozole actually stops oestrogen production, whereas Tamoxifen (the gold standard) prevents oestrogen binding to its receptor at tumour sites. Both drugs are known to have some side-effects. With Tamoxifen there is a small risk of developing endometrial cancer and increased risk of 'thromboembolic events', such as deep vein thrombosis. With Anastrozole it was known that there could be increased 'musculo-skeletal disorders' and fractures.

I had some thinking to do. In situations like this you tend to assume that you will experience the side-effects. If I didn't go on the trial, I would take a course of Tamoxifen, so my question was would weakened bones be worse than endometrial cancer? I thought not. Then there were more general questions about going on a clinical trial: am I 'typical'? (I thought not – but then probably most people think that they are not typical.) How will I feel if the cancer returns and I have been on a trial rather than taking the 'gold standard' treatment? (As the trial was comparing Anastrozole and Tamoxifen or a combination of them there was at least a fifty percent chance that I would receive the 'gold standard' treatment.) It seemed that there were no clear arguments against going on a trial and there were plenty of points in favour – not all of them altruistic. For example, on a trial I wouldn't have to pay for the drugs and I would receive free medical treatment and possibly closer scrutiny than if I were not on a trial. I might be on a new and 'better' treatment – it was very unlikely that I would be worse off. So I agreed to go on the trial.

There was a lot of explaining to do. Friends accused me of being too easily persuaded by the medical profession. 'Haven't you suffered enough?' they asked. People assumed that I was being generous and compliant. In fact, the thought that I was helping medical research was fairly low on my list of reasons for participating.

Taking the medication became part of my daily routine and I didn't think about it very much. If I became tired, or if my joints felt stiff, I did blame the trial and assumed I was on Anastrozole. But there were no significant side-effects and for five years, taking two tablets became a part of my daily routine. During this time I travelled twice to Europe – conferences followed by memorable holidays; walking along the Scottish coast, visiting the beaches of Normandy and Monet's garden at Giverny. And during this time I joined a consumer advisory panel that works closely with researchers who are dedicated in their work to find better treatments and who constantly seek the elusive cure for breast cancer.

Today, I think friends would describe me as ridiculously busy and fiercely independent – certainly leading a full life. But once a year when I return as an outpatient for my mammogram, there is that lurking fear that the cancer will return.

# My Sister's Grief

*Maureen Stahl*

It was Saturday, mid-morning, when the phone rang. It was my sister Jane.

She said, 'I've got bad news.'

My immediate thought was, *Who's gone? Mum or Dad?* Our parents were in their late eighties and frail. Every time I left them the thought passed through my mind that it might be the last time I saw them.

'It's Sarah.'

I thought, *Oh no she's lost the baby.*

Jane's next words turned the world upside down. 'She's got breast cancer.'

Tears surged to my eyes. Disbelief! Sarah, Jane's daughter, was young, vibrant, newly married, and bubbling with excitement about the imminent birth of her first baby. If someone has breast cancer surely it should be Mum or one of us daughters. We're old.

Jane elaborated on the details while I balanced on a stool at the end of the bench, my knuckles white as I clutched the phone and listened. Up until then it had been an ordinary Saturday. I was sewing, making a teddy bear from a kit. That night we were going to a dinner dance with friends. I was looking forward to it. Before the phone call life had been one way but forever after it was different.

Sarah had noticed a lump in her breast some time earlier in her pregnancy and had been told it was nothing to worry about, but it had grown rapidly. She returned to the doctor and tests were done. On Friday afternoon she went to the doctor to hear the results. She asked Jane to accompany her.

With a chill creeping through my body I listened to Jane's account of that interview.

'The doctor said, "I'm so sorry to have to tell you this Sarah but it's breast cancer," and after saying it the doctor had to wipe away tears. I felt as though I'd been struck with a sledge hammer. I was stunned but Sarah was so brave. I was so proud of her. She didn't cry. She asked, "Can you take off my breast? I can live without a breast but I don't want to die." Oh, Maureen she was so calm as she asked questions and I couldn't say a word. On the way home I said to her, "It should have been me," and she said, "No its better that it's me. I'm young and strong. My body will be able to fight it better.'

Jane's voice broke as she spoke the next words, 'People die from breast cancer.'"

When the phone call ended I went back to what I was doing but nothing was the same. A small black cloud had formed on the periphery of my vision, a small black cloud that never went away but was a constant reminder that God's in his Heaven but all's not right in the world.

For the rest of the weekend Sarah was never far from my thoughts. *She has cancer* seemed to be stamped across everything I looked at. The words echoed around everything I heard. I wondered what she and her husband, Nathan, were doing, saying, and thinking.

From the beginning of the following week Sarah's life started to read like a medical diary. On Monday she saw the oncologist.

'We'll have to bring the baby on and start treatment immediately,' he told her. 'Breast cancers in young people can be very aggressive. We need to move fast.'

On Tuesday she visited her gynaecologist who assured her the baby, at eight months, was big enough to be brought into the world safely. Arrangements were made for Sarah to enter hospital the next day for the birth to be induced.

With her never-failing ability to see the silver lining beneath the dark cloud Sarah said it was lucky they had not found the cancer when she was only a few months into her pregnancy, when she may have been encouraged to abort, and would have been faced with making a decision that no woman should have to make.

On Wednesday she arrived at the hospital but not in the excited way that she would have presented if she had been full term and going into labour naturally. The process was started and her husband, Nathan, and her family waited anxiously.

The baby wasn't ready to leave the snug comfort of the womb and resisted attempts to oust her for two days. Finally, late on Thursday evening, Lucy was expelled from her exhausted mother's womb.

'I'm so sorry, my darling,' Sarah told her. 'I promise I'll never hurry you like that again.'

On Friday morning they tried to get Lucy to suckle her mother's breasts, the only chance she would have before they started pumping Sarah's body full of dye and chemicals to perform their numerous tests, but Lucy was new, tiny, tired and not ready to suck. Sadly Sarah expressed the precious liquid before being wheeled away to undergo further invasions of her body, the joy that follows delivery cruelly cut short.

'I'm so sorry that we can't allow you more time with her to get her feeding,' the doctor was genuinely apologetic, 'but it's Friday and Monday is a public holiday. If we don't do these tests today we'll have to wait till Tuesday and it's essential to start treatment as soon as possible.'

Even the calendar seemed to be against Sarah.

The birth of this baby, the first child for Sarah and Nathan who were so keen to start a family, the first grandchild for Sarah's parents, Jane and Tony, and the first niece for Sarah's siblings, should have been the cause of joyous celebrations but the moment was shrouded in worry.

Only two people were able to enjoy the moment as they should have. Sarah's grandparents, Dolly and Frank, had not been told of the diagnosis. During the week they had been blissfully unaware of what had been going on. Jane decided that she wouldn't tell them yet, that she would simply say Sarah had gone into labour early.

Wearing an armour of resilience Jane went to their house and mustering acting skills she didn't know she possessed, she breezed in with a beaming smile and told them that Sarah had 'gone early' and they had a great-granddaughter. They were delighted by the news. Sarah was a much loved and loving granddaughter who visited them often and cheered their quiet days immensely.

'What are they going to call her?' Dolly asked.

'Lucy.'

'Oh lovely! A good old fashioned name! I like it.'

There were more questions. How heavy was she? What did she look like? Did she have red hair like her mum and Grandma? How was Sarah feeling after the birth? Jane answered with as much enthusiasm as she could muster, smiling constantly and no doubt thinking, *If only it was just like this – great news without complications.*

Dolly, who was never very keen to go out, asked Jane to take her to the shops to buy a present for the new baby. Jane obliged and took her to the local shops where they bought a doll. Dolly, who was usually quiet and retiring, beamed at the shop assistants and told them, 'I've just got a great-granddaughter, Lucy, and this is her grandmother.' She indicated Jane.

The shop assistants were enthusiastic and gave congratulations to both women. Dolly's smile was growing wider and Jane's heart was breaking.

***

Sarah began her treatment. She had chemotherapy. I knew about chemotherapy. Well, I thought I did. I'd heard about other people having it. It was a nasty business. I was soon to learn just how nasty. I knew people lost their hair. This is the obvious visible sign but hair loss hurts mainly vanity. I didn't know then about the nausea, the soreness, the aches, the lethargy, the loss of appetite and the loss of taste that also accompany it. In the weeks to come I was to hear all about these things from Jane as she watched in utter helplessness as her daughter suffered.

After the chemo came the radiation, six weeks of daily trips to the hospital, the trek there, the lengthy preparation, the momentary dose of radiation then home again. Sarah was a red head with very pale skin and I shuddered at the thought of that radiation. I visualised sunburn, something I'd often suffered through and hoped she wouldn't have anything like that to endure.

Lucy, meanwhile, grew and thrived, juggled between a sick mother, a worried father, distraught grandparents, aunts and uncles. There were plenty of loving relations and she was too young to sense the fear they were secretly carrying.

Lucy quickly learned to distinguish between 'Sick Mummy' and 'Well Mummy'. On bad days Mummy lay with her bald head on the pillow smiling weakly, but lovingly, at her daughter. On good days Mummy put on a wig, a hat or a colourful turban and they played wonderful bonding games. Lucy would gaze wide-eyed and solemn faced at 'Sick Mummy' and looked to Daddy to fulfil her needs. When 'Well Mummy' leaned over her cot she cooed, chuckled and held out her arms to be hugged. During those first months Lucy's schedule had to fit in with chemo, radiotherapy and endless trips to doctors and hospitals.

At the end of all this treatment Sarah had a lumpectomy. The doctors were hoping that the tumour had shrunk and that a lumpectomy would be all that was needed. Tests were done and everyone was hopeful that the results would be good and that a mastectomy would not be necessary. On the designated day I constantly checked my mobile phone waiting for the text message that Jane had promised to send when she knew the results.

The phone signalled and vibrated on the window ledge. I bounded across the room from where I had been ironing. The sun was shining; it was a nice day. *A day to receive good news*, I thought. I picked up the phone and read the brief message and my spirits dropped. The results were not good and a mastectomy would be needed. A cloud moved across the sun as if in sympathy with my darkening thoughts. Later I rang Jane. I expressed my disappointment and sympathy and asked how she was feeling. She told me she'd just been 'having it out with God'. I knew what she meant. Many were the times had I uttered the words, 'Why God? Why?'

Sarah had the mastectomy and some of her lymph glands removed. Jane explained to me that she would need to wear an elasticised bandage on her arm for the rest of her life. Yet another problem to contend with but she could live with that, just as she could live without one breast. She was prepared to endure all the associated difficulties as long as she could stay alive to look after Nathan and Lucy, both of whom she adored. All else was immaterial. She and Nathan had already faced the fact that there could be no more children. This saddened them as they had hoped to have a large family but Sarah felt blessed that she at least had Lucy.

She told her sisters, 'I'll just have to depend on you to have children now and Lucy will have to have little cousins instead of little brothers and sisters.'

Sarah was always cheerful. One day when I was visiting Dolly and Frank she called in with Nathan and Lucy. Dolly and Frank by this time had been told of the cancer but Jane had played it down. Sarah had a cancer but she was getting treatment and should be fine again soon was what they had been told.

It was a fine spring day. Sarah looked lovely. Her hair was growing back so her head was covered with thick tight curls, she was model slim, her skin was clear and her smile lit every part of her face. I was delighted to see her and I said, 'Hi, Sarah! How are you?'

It was an instinctive greeting but the moment it was out I wanted to take the words back. Sarah wasn't fazed. Still smiling she answered, 'Well that's a strange question these days. I suppose I could say I'm well but then I'm not really. But today is a good day, so we're pretending to be a normal family, aren't we?'

She smiled at Nathan and he smiled back but his smile didn't disguise his worry. It was etched into his features. On arrival he'd given me the customary hug of greeting and I was aware of the tension in his body. He and Sarah were very much in love. That was apparent, and always had been, to anyone who saw them together. It wasn't hard to imagine the torture he was going through.

'She tires easily,' Jane told me.

'That's not surprising,' I answered. 'After all she's been through her body is going to take a while to recover. And she's got a new baby. Babies can be very wearing.'

'Yes that's what everyone says. Lucy's a very good baby. They're lucky in that regard and Nathan is a great help to her. It's still early days I suppose.'

Sarah, with her usual optimism, said to Jane, 'I can't die. I have to get better so I can look after you and Dad in your old age, like you are looking after Nana and Pop.'

Christmas came and went and the New Year dawned. On New Year's Eve Jane and Sarah shared an intimate moment as they watched the fireworks.

'I hope this New Year is a good one. I couldn't cope with another like last year.'

'I'm sure it will be,' Jane answered, giving her a hug.

***

For the first few months things did seem to be better. It was in July that our world started to fall apart. Jane sent me an email. I could see that it was sent in the early hours of the morning, a sure sign that it was bad news – something that was preventing her from sleeping. Sarah had found another lump.

She said to Jane, 'Mum I'm so scared.'

She had good reason to be scared at the thought of going through all that treatment again. She had already made an appointment to see her doctor, who said, 'Don't panic. It could be just scar tissue.'

'Of course it's scar tissue,' we all said, trying to be positive and hoping it was.

It was Jane's birthday on the weekend and the whole family were going out for a day together. On Friday Jane rang me. She said Sarah had just got her results and it was cancer. I said, 'Oh no!'

For a moment there was silence. Then, in a strangled voice Jane said, 'Not my Sarah.' Her voice broke and through her tears she mumbled, 'I've got to go.'

The phone went dead and I just sat and stared at the receiver.

Next day was Jane's birthday. I had a card for her. I sat and looked at it. I wondered what I could possibly write in it. I couldn't say, *I hope you have a happy day.* It couldn't possibly be a happy day. I couldn't say, *I hope you have a good year.* We all knew it wasn't going to be a good year. I couldn't say, *All the best for the future.* The future was looking blacker than it had ever looked. I have never had more difficulty finding words to write.

As if in mockery the day dawned bright and clear and I wanted to scream at the sun for shining. The sky should have been dark with thunderous clouds to match the ones that were hovering over us. All day long I thought of Sarah's family and their despair. What could they possibly talk about when they all knew what was in everyone's thoughts and what they didn't want to talk about. They had their day together but it wasn't a day spent in celebration as a birthday should be. There was a sense of oppression that no one could shake.

Sarah had an appointment with the oncologist. Nathan went with her. Jane minded Lucy. The news wasn't good. They couldn't cure the cancer. He told her they could only hope to slow its progress and prolong her life. With her usual courage she faced the doctor and asked, 'How long do I have?'

With the brutal honesty his profession sometimes demanded of him he replied, 'Without treatment six months; with treatment,' he shrugged, 'who knows? Maybe five years.'

'Five years! I might just see Lucy go to school.'

With her composure intact and her usual thought for others before herself Sarah insisted that they call in at the Two Dollar Shop on the way home and buy some crayons to take home for Lucy who had just discovered drawing.

Later Sarah asked her mother, 'What do you think would be best for Lucy? If I go quickly she won't know me so well and not miss me so much. If I'm around longer she will have more memories but will hurt more when I'm gone.'

Icicles formed around her mother's heart but with immense control she replied, 'The more time she has the more memories she will have, and besides medical advances are being made all the time. A cure may be just around the corner. You must hang on and fight.'

***

The cancer had spread to other organs in Sarah's body. She got sick again, very sick. She lost weight even though we didn't think there was any excess weight left to lose. She said to her mother, 'Why did God let this happen to me?'

She wasn't the only one asking this question. I asked it many times and everyone in Sarah's family was asking it too. There was no family history of cancer; Sarah's grandparents were long lived. Sarah had never abused her body with drugs of any kind. She had never eaten to excess and become obese. She had protected her fair skin from over exposure to the sun's harmful rays. She had done everything right so why? Why? *Why?* It was a question that plagued us all in the sleepless hours of the night.

A liver function test showed that Sarah's liver had deteriorated. She was put on an anti-nausea drip and after six days of this treatment she began eating again. She told her mother, 'I must be getting a bit better because I can think more clearly now. Everything has been a bit of a blur for the last two weeks.'

'The trouble is,' Jane told me, 'when she is thinking clearly she is also able to process things and think them through and that is painful. She says she is having awful dreams.'

I think her whole family were having bad dreams. Everyone felt as though they were living in a bad dream, a bad dream they so wanted to wake up from but couldn't.

The oncologist had given them no hope but the family were not about to give up. They researched every form of cancer treatment available anywhere and discovered The Oasis of Good Hope in Mexico.

Jane told me, 'They use a holistic approach to medicine. They use the conventional methods such as chemo but they use other techniques as well. Cancer can't be cured but you can live with it and sometimes live with it for a long time. At the clinic they work hard to build up the parts of your body that don't have the cancer and keep them healthy and functioning. They also use alternative therapies; they believe in prayer and positive thinking and things like laughter therapy.' She spoke passionately. 'I know people think that it's a waste of money. It's not cheap but do we have any alternative?'

No! If your child is dying you do whatever you can even if it cripples you financially.

'But she has to be accepted into their programme first. We have faxed through her details and we have a phone interview organised. This is our last chance. They have to take her.' Jane was almost violent in her determination.

The clinic did agree to take Sarah.

Sarah told her mother, 'I want to take Lucy with me, Mum; if I'm going to die I want to have as much time with her as I can.'

'Of course you do,' replied her mother.

We could all identify with this but Sarah was ill. She

needed Nathan to care for her; he couldn't care for Lucy as well.

Jane said, 'I have to go with them.'

It was not easy for Jane to go. Another daughter, Rachel, was engaged and planning a wedding. She needed her mother. Our parents were old and Dad was unwell. They needed their daughter. Jane had a business which required her guiding hand. But Sarah's needs were greatest. Jane had to go. She had to abandon everyone else and everything else she cared about and go.

She told Tony, 'If Sarah's separated from Lucy she will fret and so much depends on attitude. She has to be positive.'

Tony agreed. 'We'll all go. We can take care of Lucy, help Nathan to look after Sarah's and give the two of them moral support.'

Tickets were purchased hurriedly, cases were packed in haste, and Sarah was prepared as best her GP could manage for the long journey.

'We're going to fight and we're going to win,' Jane told me.

She spoke with determination but her hands were trembling and tears were not far away.

There were those who thought they were wasting their time and money. Even Sarah's oncologist shook his head and gave no encouragement.

'That's the trouble with them,' Jane stormed. 'They can't see past chemo; they aren't flexible. They've been treating their patients with chemo for years and it doesn't do the job. The cancers get stronger, they make the chemo stronger, the side-effects are worse; there has to be another way and this clinic may just have found it. We have to hope.'

When your child is dying, hope is the only thing you have and you clutch it to you. You hold tight to it. You feed on it and you refuse to let it go. What parent wouldn't give their last cent and use the last of their energy if they thought it could save the child so dear to them?

\*\*\*

I visited Sarah two days before she was to leave for Mexico. I went with Jane to her house. She greeted us the way she always did, cheerfully and with a huge smile on her face. She showed us a cute little t-shirt with an owl that she had appliquéd on to it. She'd made it for a friend's son.

'I'll have to make one for you, won't I, Lucy?' She smiled indulgently at Lucy who was playing with her blocks.

It was time to go. Sarah said she would see us out. She walked to the gate with us. The car was parked about five car lengths away. Sarah walked one car length with us towards it then said, 'I'd better get back. I'm feeling a bit tired.' She kissed us and made her way slowly back through her gate and up the path and I thought, *She really is very sick.*

When she was inside laughing and smiling and being so much herself I could pretend that the situation wasn't so serious but with this small show of weakness I realised that she was much sicker than we knew.

\*\*\*

The little group flew to Mexico in September, on Sarah's brother's thirtieth birthday. It was a day they had planned to have a family dinner party. The birthday was forgotten.

Sarah's siblings accompanied them to the airport. After check-in Sarah asked them to leave, saying she didn't like prolonged goodbyes. They moved away but they didn't leave. They positioned themselves behind a pillar where they wouldn't be seen and watched from a distance. They were filled with a gnawing fear that they wouldn't see their sister alive again.

The plane took off and the hopes of all Sarah's family and friends flew with it. Sarah was very ill. She needed to be transported to the plane in a wheelchair. With the help of painkillers and the ministrations of her husband and parents she endured the long journey with never a word of complaint and always a smile for those around her.

Left at home her siblings and a group of close friends cared for the family home and worked at fundraising. Oh how they worked! A huge amount of money was raised but huge amounts of money were needed in Mexico. Treatment was not cheap.

*We complain about the cost of medical treatment at home,* Jane wrote, *but honestly we don't know how lucky we are. Every treatment here costs heaps.*

At home we anxiously awaited emails. It was a rollercoaster ride. Sometimes the news was good, Sarah seemed a little better and we were all cheered but then there were relapses and the emails reduced us to tears. There were a couple of occasions when Jane emailed that they thought the end had come but Sarah fought on.

Jane returned to Australia early in December after the sudden death of our mother. Tony and Lucy followed soon after but Sarah and Nathan remained to finish the course of treatment. Sarah was showing improvement, they reported on their return. Jane felt that maybe she had 'turned a corner'. The family were optimistic.

Christmas was fast approaching but Jane didn't want to think about it. This Christmas was going to be our first Christmas without Mum but Christmas without Sarah would not be Christmas at all. Jane's family had always been together for Christmas. Then came the news everyone at home had been waiting for.

Sarah emailed:

> Well, there's good news and then there's good news!
>
> The scan is in, and my liver is 'amazing' according to the doctor, the tumours have shrunk to small spots. They assume my lungs should be in the same kind of shape. My bone problems appear similar to last time but they take a lot longer to heal. So isn't that great?! The chemo's working so well that I should keep going with it.
>
> So finally, we have been given the OK to go home after this treatment, armed with instructions and info on how to keep working the miracle from Australia. Nath just called Qantas and we have flights on Friday night. We will be home Sunday morning - Christmas Eve! I always thought we'd make it...I will not be in great shape as it will be right in the thick of chemo side-effects but I figure everyone has seen me worse, and at least we will be there, even if my Chrissy lunch has to go in the blender.

The family prepared for a wonderful Christmas. They

were determined it would be the best Christmas ever and they would rejoice in being together and having Sarah on the road to recovery. With the widest of smiles Jane said, 'She was determined to make it home for Christmas'

Sarah and Nathan arrived home on Christmas Eve. I saw them on the evening of Christmas Day. I was surprised by how Sarah looked. She was thin and pale but she had always been thin and pale-skinned. She didn't look sick; she looked happy; more than happy – radiant. She was home with her family, somewhere she must have often feared, while in Mexico, that she would never be again. She looked better than the other family members in the room. The rest of the family looked tired. It showed in their faces and in their body language. Victims of cancer are not only the ones who are diagnosed with it. Those who are close to them suffer too.

'You look great,' I told her.

'I feel good,' she replied with her signature smile. 'I'm looking forward to the New Year. It's going to be a great one.' She looked at Nathan with Lucy on his knee and positively glowed with new purpose.

'Well it couldn't be any worse than the last one,' her brother mumbled.

But it was.

***

Everyone was happy but it was the lull before the storm. In January Sarah, Nathan and Lucy went to the coast for a short holiday.

'I just want to paddle my feet in the sea on an Australian beach,' Sarah said happily.

But she never got to do it.

The day they arrived she got a headache, a very bad headache. By the following morning it was so severe Nathan drove her home and straight to the hospital. The diagnosis was grim: a brain tumour.

The surgeons operated immediately and said they had removed it all. Sarah made a remarkably quick recovery. In a matter of days she was smiling at everyone again. She was due to go home but fluid built up on her brain and had to be drained. Fluid built up again and a permanent drain was put in. Again she overcame the obstacle but while all this was going on she was unable to continue her chemo treatments or take her medications. The cancer in its demonic fashion seized the opportunity to attack again. It was relentless. In her organs, where it had lain dormant, it flared again with ferocious intensity. The strength of her endurance amazed everyone as her body fought each fresh battering, but she was growing weaker. She fought hard, she fought bravely and she fought with a smile on her face and care in her heart for others.

'I'm not afraid of dying,' she told her mother, 'but I feel sad that it will cause all of you so much grief.'

Rachel was getting married in March. The wedding had been postponed once when there was still hope that Sarah would recover and be able to take her place as a bridesmaid. Sarah insisted they go ahead with it and she was determined to be there.

I went with Jane to visit her in hospital. I wasn't sure how I would find her but there she was sitting up in bed with a wide smile of greeting. She was wearing a woollen hat and as we talked her face became quite red.

'You look hot,' Jane said. 'Do you need to wear the hat?'

'I didn't want Maureen to have to look at my ugly bald head,' she replied.

'Oh please take it off if you're hot,' I told her.

'But I'm not a pretty sight,' she replied. 'I thought the sight of my head might upset you.'

As always she was thinking of others. At my insistence she removed her hat. All her beautiful curly, auburn hair was gone and the drainage tubes were showing like long straws beneath the stretched skin on her skull. As she had said it wasn't a pretty sight but her smile was what drew your eyes and not her bare head.

She talked about Rachel's upcoming wedding and she reminisced about good times we'd had in the past. As we laughed about a funny incident that had happened some time ago she looked at me and said, 'You must write our stories down.'

'I will,' I replied and I am fulfilling that promise.

***

Rachel's wedding was drawing closer. For a week Sarah trained for it like an athlete preparing for a race. She would leave her hospital bed for two hours, then three, then four. She would take a short trip to the cafeteria, the next day home for an hour and so on.

The day arrived and Sarah went home. Despite the pain in her frail, failing body she allowed herself to be dressed in her bridesmaid dress by Rachel and the other attendants. Jane slipped quietly out of the bedroom and leaned against the closed door, tears spilling down her cheeks,

'I can't bear to watch,' she told Tony. 'Just lifting her arms into the sleeves of the dress causes her so much pain. I can see it in her face but she's not complaining.'

'I know,' he replied, 'but you have to cheer up. This is Rachel's day. We have to smile no matter what. We can't have Rachel looking at her wedding photos in the years to come and seeing glum faces.'

It had been a long time since Sarah had been able to wear shoes but a friend had made her a pair of shoes in the softest of material to match her bridesmaid's dress.

'I love my new shoes,' Sarah beamed when she was finally ready.

Lucy was wearing a dress the same shade as her mother's.

'Look, Lucy, we have the same dresses. We match. Don't we look pretty?'

***

In a wheelchair with oxygen Sarah bravely faced the wedding guests, about two thirds of whom she had never met before. Women are vain creatures who want to appear at their best in public, especially at such occasions as weddings. Sarah was pale and frail, a mere shadow of the stunningly beautiful bride she had been so recently but she put aside vanity and smiled at everyone. She smiled throughout the ceremony when surely her heart was breaking remembering how, just three years before, she had made the same wedding vows and looked forward to a long and rewarding life ahead with her new husband. Nathan was there beside her, steering her wheelchair and taking care of her, the love apparent on his face just as clearly as it had been on his own wedding day. Sarah could have been forgiven if she had looked woeful or downcast but in true Sarah fashion she never let the smile slip from her face. She left soon after the start of the reception, exhausted.

Sarah's attendance at Rachel's wedding was one of the most courageous acts I ever witnessed and one of the most loving. It would have been easy for her to have stayed away but her presence was testimony to the great love she had for her sister and her family.

*\*\*\**

One week later Lucy celebrated her second birthday. Sarah had left the hospital. She was at home where palliative care nurses and her husband were attending to her needs. Like all small children Lucy loved balloons.

'I know what we should do for Lucy's birthday,' Sarah said. 'We'll fill the room with balloons. Imagine the look on her face when she comes in here and sees them.'

Lucy had been staying with Jane and Tony but was to come home to stay the night before her birthday. After she had gone to bed Nathan and Tony blew up hundreds of balloons so that Sarah's bedroom was quite literally filled with them.

Lucy woke early on her birthday. Daddy got her out of her cot and she ran to Mummy's room. She stopped in amazement. Sarah was overjoyed at her awed reaction. Was she thinking, *This is such an awe-inspiring moment for her – surely it will stay in her mind and she will remember me?*

The rest of the family agreed that Lucy, Nathan and Sarah should have the day to themselves. Sarah was confined to the bed so that was where they painted and built cubbies. They even had picnics meals right there on the bed. It was a special day.

The extended family came next day to belatedly celebrate the birthday. Sarah was carried to the lounge room. She smiled as she watched Lucy, in her party dress, open presents and squeal with delight. It was to be Sarah's last sight of her beloved daughter. Overcome by the exertion of the two days she slumped in her seat. Her husband carried her gently back to her bed. Jane and Tony took Lucy home with them.

At midnight Sarah died. It was two years and one week since I'd heard Jane say, 'It's Sarah. She has breast cancer.'

***

Sarah's death is not the end of her story. It was mercifully the end of her suffering but the suffering of her family was only in its infancy. While Sarah was alive they focused on her care and tried to keep bright and cheerful for her sake. With her gone, grief overwhelmed us.

How do you tell a two-year-old that she will never see Mummy again?

What do you say when your daughter jumps excitedly into the car the day after her mother's death and says, 'Go home. See Mummy?'

What do you say when a month after her mother's death your granddaughter sees a wheelchair parked outside the hospital and says eagerly, 'Mummy?'

How do you stop your heart breaking when ten months after her mother's death, after visiting her Aunty Rachel with her new baby, this little girl says, 'Mummy gone, Mummy come home soon?'

They say time heals. It's a lie. With time the bereaved family learn to present a less grief-stricken appearance but the wound is still there. Sarah's family learnt to put on a cheerful face for Lucy. Although they were always close to tears when they spoke of Sarah, they knew it would be wrong if Lucy was to always associate her mother with grief so for her they made the effort.

Life for them is bittersweet now. When they celebrate Lucy's birthday they know it is also the anniversary of Sarah's death. Rachel's wedding anniversary reminds them of Sarah's last appearance in public and the last time many of her relatives saw her. Jane's birthday reminds them of the start of Sarah's second fatal encounter with cancer. Her brother's birthday reminds them of the dash to Mexico which didn't save her life. Every new accomplishment of Lucy's, while cause for celebration, brings the sadness that her mother is not able to share it. When Lucy proudly showed the little clay pot she made at kinder for Mother's Day and said, 'This is for Mummy, I'm going it take it to the cemetery,' the tears were hard to control.

*** 

I witnessed Sarah's agony as they tried to find her veins for the IV treatments. I didn't see her suffering the side-effects of the chemo but I saw what it did to those who were there. I saw the strain on their faces, the pain in their eyes and the weariness in their bodies and I know the memories are engraved forever in their minds.

Time will never take away my sister's grief. My heart goes out to her and to her husband and her other children who are always conscious of the empty chair at their tables. I feel sad for Nathan who is now a single parent bringing up his daughter without the loving support of his soulmate and for Lucy who was robbed of her mother at such an early age. I also feel for the families of all the other Sarahs, the lovely young women who have been taken in their prime by breast cancer, and all the other Lucys, the children who have been deprived of their mothers' love and care as they grow. The sum of the suffering of breast cancer victims and their loved ones is a heavy weight in the world.

# The Funeral

*Maureen Stahl*


Grief spilled into the aisles
and through the doors.
tears fell unheeded
from red swollen eyes.
hearts ached for the loss
of a woman so young.
tributes flowed
in words rich with love
as we reflected on the life
that had been lived
and mourned for the life
that could have/
should have been.
suspended in the air
the unanswered question

Why?

# Little Blue Penguins
# Crossing at Night

*J Anne deStaic*

***For Jacqui***
*This story is written in honour of a very dear friend who died in 1999 – only four years after her diagnosis of breast cancer. She was never really free of her disease over those years but this did not stop her taking on a new job as a CEO of a large health service organisation and I doubt that many of her colleagues were aware she had cancer until after she resigned.*

*My friend found life strange and wonderful in her final months. This might have been due to her medications but I prefer to think that she finally gave full rein to her wild imagination.*

*So this account is based on my memories of her late night phone calls and the excitement of her everyday adventures.*

Up north the sky bothers me, going on and on as it does. Huge and bright, too high to touch in its middle and all faded and frayed at its edges, it is relentless. It makes me stop and wonder when I wish to do neither and I think that this is indeed its purpose and only this – to overwhelm. The overwhelming northern sky.

So I am driving south. And when I reach the end of this island there will be a sky of glory and noise, a sky so low I will walk right into it and I will be home.

I have been given six months to live which seems right because it is November now and in six months it will be May. I would not want to die in spring when the world is new, nor in summer when the world sprawls in the heat, drinks wine and laughs. Better to die in autumn, to curl up in the world while it cools.

So I will wait for autumn and while I wait I will have the lasts. The last magnolia blooming hugely in the cool spring air; the last field of jonquils and the great surprise of perfumed clouds that come with them; the last first spring rain that washes the roads clean and makes them glitter in the street lights; the last great laughing at my table set with the best of crockery and the best of friends; the last swim in the cold ocean while my bones are still solid and can pull against the waves; and maybe my last lover who will be all passion and fun.

I left early to catch the mist that wraps round the high country this time of year and now as the road rises to each hill and falls to each valley it swallows my car, damp and private. I drive through till I reach the sun and the flat low highway.

I promised my friends I would stop for food and drink, though food and drink hardly interest me anymore. But I like the conversation. I like the way the day divides itself around each meal.

The first town I come to is busy waking up and I am suddenly scared of the process of parking: the slowing, the braking, the reversing. My hands start shaking so I drive on to the next and smaller lazy town with its one main road so wide and empty and parking there is just a matter of stopping.

I get out of the car and stretch but carefully. There is a general store, one of those with a post office and books and magazines and a café off to the side. One of those where conversation is expected.

Earthquake weather. That's what she says to me, the waitress taking my order.

She stands and stares out the window so long I think that perhaps I am supposed to utter some word of dismissal and have missed my cue. She scrunches up her face as if to spy the impending event and then tucks her pen behind her ear and trots on her stilettos back to the kitchen. It is not me she is waiting for dressed like that. I look out the window. Birds land on the concrete car park, strut about for a bit and then take off. Cars pass on the road. A duck waddles around the side of the café and shakes its tail. And I think it remarkable that the waitress knows what these birds do not, that a quake is coming. She returns from the kitchen and gives me my coffee and juice and then leans on the bench near the glass case of cakes. She is staring out the door and it seems to me more likely that the birds are right.

A truck pulls off the road with a gravel flourish and birds flutter and squawk. The waitress stands up and smooths her clothes. She tilts her head and twirls a strand of hair in her fingers. The driver, young and keen, comes in the door. Earthquakes. And what would it matter to me if the world ended now in a splitting and crumbling of earth? I drink my morphine and disguise its bitterness in orange juice and heaped teaspoons of sugar. I drink my coffee. The waitress and her driver disappear out back and have not returned by the time I leave. I put the money by the till.

My bones hum in delight as their aching stops. The car flies over potholes and the map on the seat beside me shimmers in the colours of its red snaking railroads and its bold black names. The signs on the roadside sail by in yellow and gold and shout their numbers at me in the breeze that is a soft silver sigh. The thunder on the eastern hills is blue and velvet and the hills sound green in their sunshine and roar gray in their valleys. A morning sun chatters in splinters and bounces off wet bitumen. It screeches as it tears round cow sheds and farm houses and round dairy factories and abattoirs. All this noise and all this colour all down the road where all is spangle.

So here I am on the highway south, stopped at traffic lights on a dog-leg piece of road with a railway crossing close on the other side. Here I am, listening to the yellow radiance of women laughing as they walk past me, watching dogs on their leads and joggers bobbing up and down. Here I am watching the morning drifting on and the morning people bright and newly washed, and the lights change, and I take my foot off the brake and start forward. A man with a child in tow darts across the road right in front of me. I brake so hard that splinters of pain charge up my spine and hurt my breath. The man glares at me. He gestures, two fingers raised. I see the flash of a blue tattoo on the back of his hand. He has not brushed his hair nor shaved this morning. His eyes are red rimmed and dark shadowed. There is urgency in his movement and tension in his bad teeth and tattoos. There are bruises on his arms and I think, *I know you, I know your story*. His daughter beside him blushes, for it could only be his daughter, they look so alike. She wears a school uniform of sorts and will be very late for school today and soft and new and playful summer days are not for her anyway. Her father lets go of her hand and he hurries off. She stares at me and she smiles and it is a slow and graceful smile and I smile back. Her gaze is intimate. It seems to me the girl knows I am dying and wishes me well and how could that be?

They are gone. They are caught up with the happy summer people walking on the pavement. But we have something in common this man and me. We have this opiate: his damnation, my salvation

The car behind honks and the light is still green and I jerk the car forward into the empty intersection and round the angle of the road and over the railway line.

I pull to the side. I breathe and wait and the trees along the river beside the road kindly breathe and wait with me. The morning seeps again into the car and the clang of the warning bell on the railway crossing bleaches my brain of colour. The girl's face slides from memory. I finish the bottle of morphine, grateful to all those poppy flowers bleeding their white milk to give my bones their rest.

The vision of poppy fields stays with me all the way through the town and past the crystal lakes and down the soft brown desert road with its passionless mountains shifting position in the rear vision mirror. But that damn road is uneven and jarring and the pain is a red mist filling the air and I am gasping by its end. I stop again and it occurs to me that my friends were right. This was not a wise trip to make alone. I get out of the car and stretch my shoulders and arms, (these being my safe bones).

There is a roadhouse opposite and the long clumsy trucks sail into its parking bays and the drivers climb in and out of their cabs with chip wrappers and drink cans. They laugh and talk and life crackles all around them. The movement soothes. It reassures. I know this road. A gracious smooth highway.

I drive south again and the road takes me slowly to the sea, first with glimpses of a flat blue ocean and an island distinct on its long blue line; then with a clarity of waves, crested white with foam; finally with a callous wind spitting salt at the air and spitting sea foam at the road. There is a railway line to the left and a train bursts out of its tunnel like a bullet through glass, screaming and splintering the space around me and all I want now is to get home.

But there are roadworks, always roadworks, on this highway. I slow to a crawl pressed all around by other cars and the sound of machinery drowning out thought. Men work with their jackhammers; men rest on huge chunks of fractured bitumen; men smoke and talk and the sweat of their bodies is visible and horrible to me in the fading light as I creep by. The windows of my car are up but even so they leak the exhaust smell from the car in front.

I shout at those men and those cars.

I shout, I am nearly dead!

The traffic is heavy down through the gorge coming round the suburbs. Lights blink on in the cars as drivers notice the creeping dark and I turn mine on to match.

The huge wide water of the harbour is grey and solid. I turn left heading to the valley, the hills on my left and the harbour on my right and I hug the water's edge and turn right along the foreshore. There is just enough light still to see one lone rower out there in the grey water pulling against the sea. His white jacket billows in the wind and his kayak disappears behind each surge of water and he is a marvel to see. Once I would have stopped and gazed in awe at him and his strength and beauty, but today I think how arrogant is this one small man to be on such a large sea, alone. A light rain has begun to fall and it smatters my dusty car and I turn the heater on and cry for being so near to home. In the end I wish the rower well.

This road, at its end now, is cruel in its twists and bumps and my bones twist and bump to each angle and each curve but I like this piece of road stuck here at the edge of the hills with the harbour grabbing at it when the wind is high. And the wind is always high round here.

Coming up on the right I see my favourite road sign.

### Little Blue Penguins Crossing at Night

This last journey south I stop, hoping to see one of these birds amble up and out of the graceful water to waddle across the ugly road. My friend had started this ritual. She would wait for ages in her car wanting to see this little blue penguin and so anxious that if one did appear it might bumble onto the road and a car with a driver who was drunk or tired or just unaware of the world around might crash into the clumsy bird and all its innocence. But perhaps the caution is for the people in their cars who might be caught up in the maelstrom of penguins dashing for the shore, angry birds, all beaks and flapping wings.

This last journey south, sitting there alone and waiting for the bird to come I ring my friend but she is not at home, so I laugh and leave her a message. I am safe. So are the penguins. Then I remember the girl and her father at the intersection from earlier in the day. She had stared at me with knowing in her gaze and the memory is comforting. But my pain will keep no longer. And no bird appears.

I slip back onto the road and drive home in the gentle rain with the clouds humming like drums and the rain tasting of electricity and purple.

And the sky is so low I walk right into it.

# www.cancerchoice.com.au

*Delia Scales*

In September 2007, a GP told me that the biopsy of a recently discovered breast lump showed cancer. I was overwhelmed with emotion and most of it was related to my mother's experience of cancer treatment.

Diagnosed in her early forties, she refused a mastectomy and insisted on a lumpectomy. Chemotherapy made her so ill she passed out during one treatment. She was severely nauseous and could not finish the treatment. When the cancer came back several years later she agreed to radiotherapy to her left breast.

It caused acute damage to the heart, resulting in fluid in her lungs and near death. She later went on to suffer chronic and increasing swelling of the sac around the heart, called pericarditis. In her later years she was chronically short of breath. She was humiliated by her 'moon face', caused by the high dose of steroids. Her left breast looked like a piece of plastic that had melted in the microwave.

'I'm in so much pain,' she confided in me, during the last years of her life. Perhaps it was because the cancer had spread to her bones. No one knew. There was no follow up, support or symptom management from any cancer specialist.

At the age of sixty-three she went to see the GP about

being more short of breath than usual. He ordered a chest x-ray.

The next day she rang me sobbing. 'The cancer is back, it's in my lungs.'

On the long and scenic train trip up the Blue Mountains my mind churned. What was I supposed to do? When I saw how frail she was, I rang all the family and we nursed her in turns. Three weeks later she was dead.

The GP wrote five causes on her death certificate. Three were related to cancer treatment. One was breast cancer. One was cancer that had spread around her body.

Packing up her clothes I was mystified to discover two separate dress and shoe sizes in my mother's wardrobe. It was as though two women shared the one cupboard.

'Your mother had two different wardrobes,' advised a close friend. 'The fat clothes were when she was on steroids, bloated but able to breathe easily. The thin clothes were when she was off steroids and felt slim and happy, but was always short of breath.'

*How little I knew of my mother, and her chronic ill health.*

***

The GP had booked an appointment for me with a private breast surgeon for the following day. There was no discussion about public versus private cancer treatment. Meanwhile, the ghost of my mother's terrible treatment, her damaged body then eventual death, haunted me.

I was due to go overseas the following week. I had to cancel the flight, explain to the travel agent the reason, then try and claim for travel insurance refund. Then I had to cancel my shifts as a nurse.

***

The private surgeon was brisk and efficient. A second biopsy was done with a wider instrument all over my breast this time. Twenty-four hours later the results were back: cancer too big for a lumpectomy. A mastectomy was required. An appointment was made to see a plastic surgeon at the end of the week, and an operation was booked for a week's time. Further tests were also requested. It all seemed so efficient. I was impressed.

The further tests turned out to take up a full day. CT of abdomen, chest and pelvis with contrast. Nuclear med bone scans. Liver ultrasound. Chest x-ray. And numerous tubes of blood. I shook with fear during these tests, thinking, *The surgeon must have had a reason to order these tests.* The bill came to over $600, due in full on the day, no bulk billing available. It was up to me to claim what I could from Medicare. I was shocked, and had to borrow the money.

The visit to the plastic surgeon was worse. The out of pocket cost was $3,500. At least she gave me an upfront quote.

Then the hospital rang me the day before the operation was due. 'Your private health rebate does not cover the costs. Bring $5,000 before the operation, cash or Eftpos, or the operation can't go ahead. No cheques accepted.'

I spent the day of my mastectomy borrowing the money, running to the bank to take out the cash, and fighting with my private health fund. I had missed out on the right level of cover by two months. There was nothing they could do. I also posted a letter of resignation to work that morning, I had no sick leave and could not see myself going back to work for some time. I arrived at the hospital late and distressed. All I could think about was being indebted beyond my ability to repay the loans I was accumulating. I had a large mortgage I was paying on my own. How was I going to continue to make the repayments?

The surgery was successful and the plastic reconstruction done at the same time was wonderful. I literally went into theatre with a breast and came out with one. With a shirt on, you would not know that that an operation had taken place. My self-confidence was revived. Someone understands how important it is to put something back for women with breast cancer, instead of continuously taking away their health and looks and self-confidence.

Two days after the operation was over I rang an estate agent, and put my house up for sale. I'd never been in debt in my life, and couldn't go on borrowing from my boyfriend. I could see the cost of breast cancer treatment was going to be enormous. I didn't consider getting a second opinion. Going back to the GP, getting another referral to another specialist and going through another set of tests, diagnosis and treatment plan was unimaginable. My emotions were like a wild storm. All I could do was get through each day.

The private surgeon cross-referred me to a private oncologist who worked in her clinic. He was a cold, disinterested man, who announced that I needed three months of chemotherapy and five years of Tamoxifen, in the same tone that you would expect someone to announce that the stock market had dropped a few points. I was shattered, and walked out of his office in a daze.

\*\*\*

My thoughts went back to my mother, and her experiences of cancer treatments. The doctors told her nothing about the side-effects and how to manage them. Her family didn't get any information either, and sometimes things ending up taking an unexpected turn.

My mother had heard from girlfriends that chemotherapy made your hair fall out, and was determined not to be left looking unattractive. She decided to buy a wig in Sydney, before chemotherapy started. She took me along for company. I was a rebellious teenager at the time, with short scruffy hair, torn clothes and an angry attitude. We argued in the car, all the way from Newcastle to Sydney. Why did I have to be so rebellious? Why did she break up the family when I was five? Why did I blame her for everything? Why was she so obsessed with money and social status?

We only stopped arguing when we got to Sydney. We both walked into the wig shop. Rows of brown, blond and black hair pieces, sat on fake heads along the shelves. While I stared in horror, an effeminate man came out, and walked up to me. He started to assess my head size and shape and the colour of what was left of my hair.

'I think I've got something that will be perfect,' he announced, and turned to walk off. My mother and I looked at each other, then burst into laughter. It was one of the few bright moments we shared during that time.

\*\*\*

I went back to see the private oncologist one more time and agreed to treatment. The benefits of chemotherapy for my type of cancer and the side-effects were never discussed with me. It was only after pressing from my boyfriend that the private oncologist pulled out an expensive pen and scribbled a few words on a piece of paper. He pushed it towards me with a distasteful manner, as though I did not have the right to ask him these questions.

> *Nausea, alopecia (temporary hair loss), mouth ulcers. Use Difflam mouthwash. If temperature goes over 38 degrees, go to hospital.*

That was the total education I ever received about chemotherapy.

The officious young doctor's nurse who ran around doing phone calls and paperwork weighed me, measured my height, then gave me an appointment time and date to start the treatment. The breastcare nurse spoke to me for ten minutes.

'Breast cancer is a curable disease,' she announced cheerfully. I was given a handful of brochures from the Cancer Council and a booklet from a breast cancer organisation called *My Journey*.

'Here's my card. If you have any problems, call me.'

I stood outside this private clinic, with no one to talk to, and a bag of booklets. I threw them all in the bin, and drove to my best friend's house in Geelong.

'They ruined my mother's life,' I sobbed. 'I will never forgive the doctors for what they did to her.' I cried in my best friends arms. She held me tightly, then sat up all night with me, drinking, feeding me food and listening patiently to the terrible story of my mother's treatment at the hands of private doctors. I didn't know where the grief and pain came from. I had buried it for years. It was like crying razor blades. Or shards of ice.

I turned up to the private hospital a week later with no idea what to expect, very fearful and highly anxious. The first thing the hospital secretary said was, '$750 upfront for the overnight stay, plus $350 upfront for the chemotherapy.' I rang my boyfriend, and he paid for me.

My best friend, also my lifesaver, came with me. She had talked to me continuously throughout this time, about cancer, its impact, the treatment and how to manage it. Every day she talked about money, how partners and family are affected, and how others coped. She is a trained nurse. She had also done postgraduate study in a cancer ward, in the public health system. Without her, I would never have made it through that dark time of my life.

I sat in the oncology day ward for half an hour before a nurse even spoke to me. She was busy; there was only one nurse working with six to eight patients. One woman was sobbing in front of me. It was her first day too, and she had no one to sit with her. Another woman took off a scarf to reveal a bald head, covered in fluff. It looked horrendous, like something from a Nazi death camp. Another woman vomited into a bowl.

Finally the nurse came over, tossed a Cancer Council brochure on chemotherapy in my lap, and inserted a cannula in the back of my hand. The chemotherapy made me ill straight away. My head felt as though it had been hit with a baseball bat. I was instantly and violently nauseous.

'Why haven't you given her anti-nausea medication?' I could hear my friend querying the nurse. Afterwards,

I staggered up to the toilet, and was shocked to find my urine was red.

'Is it blood?' I asked my best friend. 'Is that the cancer?'

'Of course not, it's the type of chemotherapy you have been given. It turns people's urine red for the first couple of days. The nurse should have told you that.' I could tell my friend was irritated but I was too ill to ask why.

I was taken up to a single room in the surgical ward of the private hospital and left. I was very ill. My best friend had to go. I watched her solid, comforting figure walk off up the carpeted corridor with a sinking heart.

I was wide-awake the entire night. I had severe stomach cramps, overwhelming nausea and a confused, woolly head. Despite ringing repeatedly, no doctor was called to review me. The nurses came into the room, stared blankly at me, then walked off. One basic anti-nausea drug was given overnight, and one small dose of Valium was given in the morning. Neither alleviated the symptoms at all.

In the morning the surgeon and oncologist swept into the hospital and passed through my room.

'We all know that people who are anxious have more nausea after chemotherapy,' the surgeon announced pompously.

'I'm sorry the medication affected you in this way,' remarked the oncologist stiffly.

They swept off and I was discharged quickly, or pay another $750 upfront. No one wrote a script for nausea, or stomach cramps, or dizziness. Or even let me know that such medications even existed.

I lay on the sofa at home desperately ill, for days on end. My best friend kept ringing me.

'Call the doctor. Get a script from him. You're paying all this money. It's their job to look after you.'

Finally I rang the doctor's nurse who told me, 'Oh that's typical chemo, get used to it.' She did agree to get the oncologist to fax a script for a basic anti-nausea drug to my chemist. It did nothing. My friend continued to ring every day, and faxed me a list of anti-nausea drugs.

'You just need the right combination of drugs to manage. Ring them again.'

I gave up, battling the lack of interest at the private. But I did go to the local GP. I took the list of drugs my friend had sent me, and the GP rang Canberra to get approval for a drug designed especially for chemotherapy nausea. It was very expensive; one script got you four tablets. It also helped the nausea. The other thing I did was stop eating. I figured you can't throw up if you don't have anything in your stomach.

I lost fifteen percent of my body weight during chemotherapy, going from a size twelve to a size eight. Despite repeated complaints to the oncologist and the nurses about not being able to eat, and having to buy a new wardrobe because I had lost so much weight, no one showed any interest. Every visit was the same. The doctor's nurse rushed into the room, and said, 'Are you alright? Good.' The oncologist quickly checked the blood results then sent me off for more chemotherapy.

I was at the GP every week, getting scripts for anti-nausea drugs. The GP bravely battled with the Canberra bureaucrats to get me the drug.

'Why does she need it?'

'Because she's sick from chemotherapy'

'But she's just had a script'.

'She needs another one'.

No sooner had I paid the private oncologist $160 for each visit, then I paid $350 for each chemotherapy session, $50 for their small amount of basic anti-nausea drugs that were useless, then $60 for the GP's visit and $32 for each script of Ondansetron.

As chemotherapy continued I became anorexic. Even the shopkeepers looked at me sadly and said, 'Something's wrong.' They had far more insight than the private doctors or their nurses. I crashed my car, I was so confused. Nausea overwhelmed me day after day. I stared at the clock continuously waiting for the next anti-nausea tablet. My mouth went white from lack of blood, and became dry and painful. My skin went dry and cracked. The Ondansetron caused severe constipation. I didn't use my bowels for a week, then bled from straining.

My boyfriend would come in from work every day and look at me lying on the sofa, white-faced and nauseous.

'It will be a great day in my life when I come home and you are not ill,' he said sadly.

I had asked a number of women during chemotherapy if they were left ill and without any help on their first night of treatments. All of them said they had the same experience as mine, left ill, despite repeated requests for assistance. On the final day of chemotherapy, I asked one of the nurses why this was happening.

'The doctor never writes any drugs, so we have nothing to give the patients. It happens all the time.'

After treatment was over, I rang the breastcare nurse, and told her that I was given no chemotherapy education, was left ill all night in hospital after the first treatment, then given no anti-nausea drugs during the entire treatment, despite ringing and complaining to the doctor's nurse.

'That's not my problem,' she responded. 'It's the hospital's problem.'

'Well, I think you should know what's going on,' I replied.

'Everyone has a different reaction to chemotherapy,' she replied soothingly, 'and every treatment can be different.'

She sent me a brochure from the Cancer Council on moving on after cancer treatment.

After chemotherapy was over, my health collapsed. Infection after infection overwhelmed me. Vomiting from gastro, sudden and severe urinary tract infections, systemic fungal infections, chest infections – all severe, drawn out and very slow to recover from.

My front teeth rotted, had to be pulled out, a plate organised and after rounds of antibiotics, a new tooth put in.

'Oh, chemotherapy always causes dental decay,' said the dentist.

I was spatially confused and collapsed frequently. After one severe fall I broke ribs. I had to bind my chest up for six weeks while it healed.

'Chemotherapy given to people under the age of fifty always causes osteoporosis,' remarked the chemist, and suggested I get a script for Fosamax, a drug normally given to old people.

I had changed to a woman oncologist in the private clinic, thinking that she might have a more sympathetic manner.

'We are really pleased you had your chemo,' she announced cheerfully.

I told her about the severe fatigue, dizziness and confusion. I also had strange symptoms, like heat waves, painful and sudden urinary tract infections, and inability to sleep.

'That's great. Your cancer is estrogen receptor positive. The chemo has stunned your ovaries and put you into menopause.'

I stared at her shocked. 'What are you talking about? Chemotherapy? Menopause?'

She wrote me a script for Tamoxifen, and gave me a brochure as well.

'It will make you put on weight, that's all. There are no other side-effects.'

Tamoxifen was like a fog descending over me. I couldn't hear, or think properly. I developed flu-like symptoms, freezing cold one minute, boiling hot the next. Heart palpitations were intense and frightening. And a terrible pain in my left hip, which had started up after chemotherapy, became sharp and agonising. It was as though a burning poker had been stabbed into my hip. I was ill all the time.

One day my boyfriend looked at me, hobbling around the house, pale, ill and miserable.

'You're not prolonging your life,' he remarked. 'You're living a death. Seriously, you need to take a look at what this treatment is doing to you.'

I told the oncologist I was not going to take Tamoxifen anymore.

'You're the kind of person who will be dead in ten years,' she shot back.

I decided to have the other breast removed. One in five of my mother's family had died of cancer. I had always wanted both my breasts removed. No GP had ever believed me.

Before the second mastectomy I was surprised to have to go through all the full body scans again. There was no cancer; this was an elective operation.

Eighteen months after I had been referred to this private clinic, I had a chance conversation with a public hospital nurse, who worked in a public chemotherapy day unit. I explained my chronic ill health after chemotherapy.

'That sounds very unusual,' she remarked.

I told her about my dramatic weight loss during treatment, and how nobody seemed interested.

'Did they reweigh you before each chemotherapy treatment?' she asked.

'What do you mean?' I replied.

'It's compulsory where I work to reweigh all patients before each chemotherapy session,' she replied. 'If the patient loses more than ten percent of their body weight then the doctors have to adjust the dosage …'

It was as though a piece of ceiling had fallen off, and crashed on to my head. I sat there shocked to my core. I was never reweighed by anyone during my eighteen months at this private clinic, where I had spent $15,000. I had never had any kind of a health assessment. No one had ever acted on my repeated complaints about chronic ill health, failure to recover, weight loss, infections, bone and joint pain. The doctor's nurses had just stared blankly at me in-between doing clerical work, and parroted the same phrase: 'All patients react differently to cancer treatment …' There were no information booklets, no referrals to nutritionalists. No education. Nothing.

On my final visit to the clinic I asked one of the doctor's nurses who was in charge.

'What do you mean?' she asked, vacant-faced as usual.

'Who is in charge of cancer treatments at this clinic? Patients are meant to be reweighed prior to each chemotherapy dose. I was never reweighed. Who is in charge of chemotherapy here?'

'This is not related to the hospital. These are private doctors' rooms.'

My best friend finally told me that she thought my care at the private clinic was dreadful, but also typical of private cancer treatment.

'At public hospital, we couldn't start chemotherapy before giving each new patient an hour of education. We had to do a full set of vital signs and reweigh the patient before each treatment. I was shocked when I saw what they were doing to you. I told you to go to the public sector halfway through your chemotherapy. But you were so ill, and I thought I'd better not push it.'

I put in an FOI application to see my medical records. The drug chart had height, weight and body surface area printed on each drug chart. In all but one, that information was left blank. The hospital nurse had ticked off a checklist about my health before each chemotherapy treatment. But none of those questions had been asked of me. There were no health assessments, no reference to my chronic ill health, the dramatic weight loss, the joint pain, the chronic infections.

I looked up the private hospitals section of the

department of human services, and sent in a letter of complaint about my treatment. Weeks later someone responded, and a month later I made an appointment to see a bureaucrat. I took in copies of all my records, and what I could find about what should happen when people have cancer treatment.

'This is not right,' I said. 'I paid these people all this money and they neglected to give me basic care.'

'We'll look into it,' they assured me.

I later found out that private hospitals refuse to supply the same information on patient numbers, medical procedures undertaken and strategies that have been successfully implemented to improve *safety* for patients, that the public hospitals are forced to.

'Every time DHS tried to get more information from private hospitals, they just clam up,' said a retired bureaucrat. 'And then you get medical, business and political groups on the phone, pressuring you to back off. It's just not work investigating them.'

Even the secretary at DHS knew more than I had when I was first diagnosed with cancer.

'Oh, I would never go private for cancer treatment,' she said, 'after what I've heard people say about it'.

A year later, and after numerous phone calls, DHS finally wrote back to say that the problems with the private hospital were now fixed. They advised me that DHS had no jurisdiction over private companies, like the private clinic.

A month later the private hospital's nursing manager rang me and asked, 'Would you be interested in attending a meeting, so we can see how you are going?'

As soon as I had agreed, a secretary rang to say the doctors from the clinic would be attending. Frightened of a confrontation, I brought along my boyfriend, and another male friend.

'We would like to tape this meeting,' was the first comment from one of the private doctors.

I was astonished. 'Why would you want to do that?' I asked. I realised that what had begun as an informal request by a nurse manager for a casual chat with an ex-patient who had complained about her treatment to the health department had been transformed into a medical review gathering information for legal implications.

'No,' I replied. 'That's not what this is about'.

My complaints about my treatment were dismissed out of hand. Reference was made to my emotional state. The doctors from the clinic then got up as a group, and swept out of the room together. I couldn't believe I had trusted these people with my health.

But the worse was to come.

I started going to a public hospital for follow up appointments.

'What did you have chemotherapy for? You only had Grade One Cancer.'

'But, it was recommended to me ...'

The public oncologist showed me a software system on the internet, called Adjuvent.com. It calculated reduction in death over a ten year period for people diagnosed with breast cancer and given treatment. For my age, stage and size of breast cancer, the reduction in death from breast cancer for chemotherapy was 2%

The public oncologist also ordered blood tests at every review.

'What is this?' I asked.

'It's standard to do bloods monitoring breast cancer

tumour markers for patients having follow up reviews for the first five years post diagnosis.'

I had never seen these blood tests before. No one at the private clinic had done them for me.

The breastcare nurse there was sympathetic and intelligent. She spent an hour with me, chatting about whatever I wanted to talk about.

'We often get private patients come to the public system after they have spent a lot of their money but have not been given support or follow up.' She gave me no brochures from the Cancer Council. She just listened to me.

I went home and told my boyfriend. He looked at me, and said quietly, 'You've got to get these people. They've fucked you. And they will keep on doing to others what they have done to you until someone stands up to them.'

'Private doctors are a law unto themselves,' warned several senior oncology nurses I spoke to. 'They don't want their patients to be educated. They don't want a team approach to healthcare. The private hospitals only exist to give them what they want. They know that if the private doctors don't get their way, they will take their private patients to another hospital, and they will lose the business.'

I created a website www.cancerchoice.com.au about my personal experiences. I then went to work as a nurse, in the public health system, with cancer patients. I read everything I could find about what was supposed to happen when people had cancer treatments.

I then created www.cancerquestions.com.au about all the policies and procedures, standards of care and best practices currently recommended for the management of patients having cancer treatments.

I will lobby for an enquiry into the private health system. I believe standards of care for cancer patients should be made a legal requirement.

According to the DHS website, the majority of cancer treatment is now conducted in the private health system.

The September 2011 issue of the Breast Cancer Network of Australia's magazine, *The Beacon*, ran a story on the cost of breast cancer treatment.

The Consumers Health Forum of Australia has publically raised the issue of over servicing of pathology testing causing unnecessary financial hardship to sick people.

The Medical Fraud Unit has been closed down after lobbying from medical groups claiming their investigations have been biased.

# Penumbra

*Kerrin O'Sullivan*

*In order for the light to shine so brightly, the
darkness must be present*
*– Francis Bacon*

It begins with a shadow. And in the end a shadow
remains.

But I am getting ahead of myself. For there was much
before that – unknown to me as it was, at the time. As
the doctor said, it had to have been there for much
longer. Undetected, growing. An insurgent advancing in
peaceful territory. Even on an x-ray, invisible.

Invisible? Perhaps not. Camouflaged, perhaps. But
there nonetheless – hidden, secretly thriving, mocking
machines and medicos alike.

In contempt of regular checks and clean screening
results, my cells were in anarchy. I felt vividly well,
oblivious to the fact that my body was moving me into
the world of illness. A clandestine yet efficient betrayal.
I was slipping into the world of the unwell. Perversely,
only the treatment was to make me feel poorly, not the
illness.

Breast cancer. That is how it was for me.

\*\*\*

Rewind the footage of memory, recount the events as they unfold, seek an order from chaos.

***

On a bright December morning, I am in a hotel at which I have never stayed before, celebrating an anniversary. The room overlooks a lazy brown river and the city beyond it is waking. I am watching a BBC report from Afghanistan. On the screen, a foreign correspondent is speaking earnestly, emphatically, into the camera. Frowning Afghani men in striped robes and turbans surround him. Beside a tank, a British soldier in battle fatigues is perched on a miniscule camp stool, his large body slumped in a language of defeat, weeping.

I find a lump. There is no uncertainty. Under my fingertips is a hard marble-sized lump. My appetite for breakfast evaporates. Outside, the sky appears to have clouded over, ever so slightly.

***

No debate.

The doctor agrees there is a lump. I am directed to radiology for X-rays. The room has four walls of green-grey hue, and a machine. And a therapist who attends, then leaves to shelter from the spray of radioactive rays. A pattern to be repeated many times in the months ahead. There is a gloom in the room that seems not entirely related to the quality of the light.

Waiting rooms are well-named. Time is not of the real world; the description is apt. One waits. A nurse emerges to speak to me. She inhales deeply, looks into my eyes.

'It is essential that you keep your appointment for the ultrasound tomorrow.'

A Brechtian pause.

I nod.

'*Essential*. Do you understand?'

I nod again. I understand.

The ultrasound is also in a room with green-grey walls, or has my illusory memory fabricated that? Downstairs, underground. Like a cubist bunker: dim, airless, rectangled. I seem to have entered a subterranean world of artificial light. Fluorescent tubes, halogen sunlight.

The gel is cool on my skin, its texture delicious like the jellied fingerpaint of pre-school. The technician peers at the screen, brow furrowed, perplexed. Some amorphous part of me swirls on the screen. The technician leaves, returns with a specialist. Each points at the screen in turn, shadows morph into shapes that form and re-form. In hushed tones, they deliberate. There is a folding and unfolding of white-coated arms. I am an audience of one in the wings of a darkened theatre. A deferential spectator, yet ... centre stage. The two bespectacled magicians perform a duet, juggling ideas, pointing, gesticulating in the twilight glow cast by the monitor. I strain to hear. It is as if someone has found the mute button and pressed it. I leave no wiser, with instructions to return to my doctor.

I find myself in a café near the hospital. A café exceptional only for its blandness. I have become a figure in an Edward Hopper painting.

The report does not sit well with the doctor. She asks me to return in the afternoon to see an oncologist for another opinion.

'It is not cancer,' he beams decisively and repeats the

good news. He outlines an hypothesis about ductile inflammation and writes a script for a hefty regimen of antibiotics. His kind eyes and authority reassure me.

A week passes. I follow the prescribed regimen of medication and go back. The lump has enlarged, not diminished. I feel like a yo-yo on a tight string. Apple green leaves flutter playfully on the branches of a mighty elm outside the window. Shadows of doubt flicker in the speckled summer light.

The good doctor volunteers no hypothesis. Later I realise he has put together the pieces of the puzzle. He knows. But now, naively, I do not realise this. I ask no questions; I am like an extra in a play without a speaking part. My fate is decided. We will meet in the operating theatre. The lump must come out.

***

The surgery is done at an hour early on a Friday morning when I am usually at the market, eyeing watermelon, deliberating over Sicilian olives, resisting a wheel of triple cream brie. The assisting doctor talks to me as I lie on the operating table, clasps my free hand with her warm one while the anaesthetist inserts tubes into the other. An act of gratuitous kindness. It soothes.

Days pass. Somewhere, in a lab, a pathologist examines tissue. Then one morning, while trawling the CBD in peak hour, my mobile rings, sounding the belly-dancing music a daughter has mischievously installed.

It is the surgeon; the results are in. I have cancer. Proven, invasive.

Traffic lights change from green to red. Cars slow, stop, move on. A truck belches black fumes into the urban ether. A cyclist draws up alongside my window, our eyes connect. I have the sense he is a mirage. He moves forward, yet I feel as if I am rolling backwards. I am calm, vacantly mindlessly calm. My right leg starts to tremor itself into a violent shake. I try to still it, but cannot.

There is more surgery and there is radiotherapy daily for six weeks. I resolutely do whatever I am told. I become an automaton in a medical sci-fi. Obedience, submission, faith in the expertise of the experts. Raw, blind faith.

Doctors and nurses prod my body and probe tissue. Medical students peruse, engrossed. Technicians measure angles to guide the assailing electromagnetic rays. They draw on my body with blue felt pens, then tattoo tiny stars in indelible ink to define the field of radiation. Strangers, all.

Red lines of lasers illuminate boundaries on white skin in rooms painted – oh yes indeed – green-grey. I lose all inhibitions, all vestiges of the private self I once was. Any frivolous notion of propriety I may have believed I possessed over my own body is dispensed with. I have been inducted involuntarily into the world of the unwell. A Sontag-esque nightside of life eclipses my days.

At last I emerge blinking from the underworld of the ill and re-enter what a fellow traveller once called 'the unshadowed world of the well'. I embrace health with gusto and my mind curls back to a life before cancer like a whisper of smoke from a votive candle.

Still the spectre of the cancer returning, haunts. A sun-spot on the sun's surface of health. A penumbra on the future.

And yet, for a shadow to exist, there must be light.
The light draws the eye.
The shadow fades and hope conquers fear.

# On First Hearing of Jane's Cancer

*Greg Pritchard*

this world, like the rivers that cover it
will flow inexorably, and in the push
things of beauty are destroyed

i can offer no consolation
my metaphysics does not allow respite
no afterlife, no soul, no optimism

I can only appreciate beauty when I see it
treasure it when it is in my grasp
and lament its loss

# Scared

*Greg Pritchard*

putting sheets on the bed
i am filled with an overwhelming sense of loss.
our history floods my eyes
and i can only think of you
in this bed, a smile like rose petals to greet me.

embarking on a new affair
i am torn by this shared history,
by the pain I feel each time i
see your beautiful face
or some asks how you are.
how you are.
as though you could be anything but scared.
as though we could be anything but scared.

# Third Leg of the Triathlon

*Jennifer Sutton*

The third leg of my triathlon, radiation therapy, is finally in sight, and I tell myself, yet again, *Don't be too smug*. Compared to a diagnosis of cancer, being told it's spread to my lymph nodes and a radical mastectomy a week later, then eighteen weeks of gruelling chemotherapy, six weeks of radiation therapy seems practically a doddle. But now's not the time to let my guard down. Cancer is clever – cunning even. The slightest hint of complacency and it'll be back.

Not today. I'm ready for radiation therapy.

Bring it on.

\*\*\*

I inch down Dandenong Road, steadfastly stuck in the morning peak hour traffic, feeling my blood pressure rising as I realise, as I stop at yet another red light, that I'm going to be late. I sit there and absently gaze into the distance and see the tall jacarandas instantly recognisable in summery purple, and they remind me that Christmas is close and the milestone I set when I was first diagnosed a lifetime ago – to still be alive to celebrate it – is tantalisingly within reach.

'This is the eight o'clock news. Fine weather with an expected top of a very pleasant twenty-six degrees. The top story this hour – outrage, as a Melbourne hospital confirms it's been routinely treating domestic pets at its radiation clinic on weekends. But more on that story later. First—'

I swing into the hospital basement car park, rapidly plunging down the concrete ramp. The radio annoyingly cuts out before I can find out which hospital they're talking about.

*** 

I quickly glance again at my watch, confirming I'm already late as I emerge from the car park, mole-like, directly into a hubbub that is the hospital ground floor. Instantly disorientated, I wander around in a fog of confusion and anxiety, trying to get my bearings, not sure where I should be. My appointment with Caroline Parkinson – my radiologist, the next in a long line of medical experts – was at eight-fifteen, which was five minutes ago. I'm not even sure I'm in the right building.

It's a big public city hospital, so big there are even maps and street signs. I hungrily look for any indication of where the radiation therapy unit might be and hurriedly dash along a long corridor that is already so crowded with patients and hospital staff that if I came across anyone I actually knew, we'd have to move over to the side to get out of the traffic to talk. After the comforting atmosphere of the Breast Clinic, my makeshift home for the past six months, this place is strange and foreign and feels like I've moved to the city from a small country town. I know if I got lost here I'd never be found.

Finally, I stumble into the radiation therapy reception area, ten minutes late, already worried I've somehow jinxed this leg of my treatment by not being punctual and rush up, almost throwing myself at the reception desk. The two uniformed women behind greet me in unison.

'Good morning,' they sing. 'And who are you here to see?'

'I'm Jennifer Sutton,' I breathlessly announce. 'I'm here to see Caroline Parkinson.' I wait, hoping I've stated a name that's familiar and my orienteering efforts are rewarded with a positive response.

'Have a seat over in the waiting area,' smilingly instructs the younger one, 'and could I ask you to fill in this paperwork, and could you bring it back over to me when you're finished? That would be great. Here, take a clipboard, that should make it a little easier.'

I look around to find a seat, settle down in a grubby grey vinyl chair, and get on with filling out the various forms. When I'm done, I settle back and glance around, surveying the scene. At least there's no pets in here, I muse, smirking to myself. Given the story on the radio this morning I wouldn't be at all surprised to see a Dalmatian sitting opposite me.

When my son Christian – who's now ten – was little, he had the normal small boy fascination with public toilets and would rate each one he went into. I reckon I'm getting the same with hospital waiting rooms. This one's large, dilapidated and feels as welcoming as an airport waiting area. An eclectic mix of vinyl chairs and sofas, coffee tables and out of date, much thumbed-through magazines, matches the mix of people transiting through. My rating? I give it minus ten.

There's a wider cross section of the community here than at the Breast Clinic, and most of the patients are much older. I feel strangely out of place. Instead, I should be a support person, caring perhaps for an elderly aunt who should be here, sitting next to me. Clearly I'm not supposed to be the one who's sick; ask me back in another thirty years. To make matters worse there's men here too and I'm not at all sure I want to be treated near them.

It all seems a very long way away from what I've been used to. Up until now, all I've known is the Breast Clinic where the only patients are women, all of us battling the same disease – breast cancer. More than just providing treatment, it was a place of refuge. Small and personal, where the receptionist knew my name. Even the chemo ward had a family atmosphere and was more like a lounge room than a sterile hospital treatment room. In it would sit six of us, female patients of various ages and backgrounds all battling the same shared tormentor, each patient in a recliner lounge facing into the middle of the small room and we would easily chat while we each received treatment. It wasn't hard to make friends, instantly bond, all of us in the same boat, confronting and supportive all at the same time.

Looking around the radiation therapy waiting area I realise, with a jolt, that I've left home and I'm now well and truly on my own.

'And next up, how to lose weight by turning household cleaning chores into a fabulous work out regime …' the morning television presenter inanely giggles from the wall mounted television behind me. I reach over to pick up a magazine and absently flick through, bored and realise it's going to be a long wait, and then turn to rummage through my handbag searching for my mobile to text my friend Fiona:

Waiting at radiation reception. Ask me ANYTHING
about Brad and Angelina.

Finally, I hear my name called and look up to see a young,
twenty-something tall, dark haired attractive female
nurse in standard navy blue hospital uniform standing
on the far side of reception, surveying the assembled
patients to see which one of us stands up. I quickly gather
my things and hurry over.

'Hi, Jennifer, I'm Sally,' she says, smiling. 'I'll take you
on a quick tour before you see the doctor and then we'll
start. So have you had radiation therapy before?'

'Nope, this is the first time, though I've known several
people who've gone through it,' I say, trying to hide my
nervousness.

'Alright, let's start. You're coming here for six weeks,
aren't you? Well you come in every workday, usually
around the same time,' she says as she turns and guides
me through a doorway into an area with change cubicles.
'You come into one of these cubicles and get changed into
a robe. Just remove all your clothes from the waist up,
and remember to take your clothes with you when you
leave. You can put them in one of these carry baskets.' She
points to a stack of baskets nearby that look like they've
been stolen from the twelve items or less checkout at the
local supermarket. 'Take your basket with you when you
go down to the treatment room.'

I try to absorb the information, feeling I've already lost
track, and certain I'll find when I return that I've failed
to comprehend the most obvious of instructions. If only
I could get her to write it all down – anything to help my
poor chemo brain retain at least some of the necessary
information.

'Then when you finish your treatment for the day, come back here, get changed and you store your robe in one of these pigeon holes over here in this cupboard.' She points to a series of small nooks with names neatly labelled underneath and I realise I'm well and truly in the hospital system, affirming yet again that I really am sick.

'Come through and I'll show you where you'll be treated.'

We proceed on and turn to walk down a long, wide corridor, dodging a steady stream of people walking towards us, a mix of harried hospital staff and patients including, inexplicably, numbers of elderly men, all dressed in bathrobes, walking along bare-legged, and each holding a shopping basket.

Along the corridor I see there are work cubicles interspersed between small offices, where hospital staff are congregated, either peering intently at computer screens or standing in small groups earnestly discussing something – an important patient issue or possibly just the cricket. It all adds to the generally busy feel of the place. As we continue on the nurse gestures to a small passageway ahead leading off the main corridor.

'Treatment Room Three is down here,' she instructs and we veer off into the passageway, stopping as we go in the doorway of a large windowless room to the side that looks more like the control centre of NASA – with a bank of computers positioned around its perimeter – than the hospital treatment room I was expecting.

'This is where we monitor your progress,' she says. Two youngish women, who are sitting at the computers, look up and, smiling, wave to me.

'This is Simone and over on the side is Sonya. They'll be watching you on their screens while you're having your treatment so you know at least you're not alone in there.'

Just as I wonder where *there* is we set off again, proceeding further along the narrow passageway and turn, immediately entering what I realise must be the treatment room. It's a large, brightly lit, cavernous white space, instantly much cooler than the main corridor and there, in the middle of the room, taking up half the space is a huge, dark grey brooding machine. There's a low, white treatment bed positioned in front of the machine and suspended above the bed, arching over it, a large, heavy grey metal arm, shaped like a donut that's been cut in half.

'So this is where you have your treatment. It only takes a couple of minutes, but the setting up takes quite a while. Today we're going to start mapping, drawing the grids we base your treatment on. So now, if you don't have any questions, I'll take you around to meet the doctor and when you're finished seeing her, we'll start.'

I can't summon any questions, too dumbfounded to find my voice, scared stiff, worried about what they're going to do to me next, and petrified that the next leg of treatment is going to be my ultimate undoing.

We wander back out of the treatment room, up the passageway and continue further along the main corridor to stop abruptly in front of a bank of utilitarian offices where the nurse deposits me, gesturing for me to sit in one of three metal-framed visitor's chair positioned along the wall.

I hear one of the doors open and look up to see a female head, gopher-like, popping out from one of the offices and hear in a soft American accent, 'Jennifer?'

'Yes?' I question as the woman fully emerges, hand stretched out in front, saying as she shakes mine, 'Caroline Parkinson.'

I meekly follow her back into the office, arriving surprisingly quickly, and realise her office is the same size as a postage stamp. She's my age, mid-late forties, tall with long dark hair. She's dressed in a dark, slim-fitting dress and as I seat myself in the visitor's chair positioned at the edge of her desk, I have the uncontrollable urge to peek down to check out her shoes, realising she's incongruously glamorous, strangely out of place in the cramped dreary public hospital office. She also immediately comes across as relaxed and devoid of normal medical expert formality, and I instantly like her. She takes me through the preliminaries in checking my medical history.

Then without further ceremony, she says, 'Okay, let's examine you.'

I move over to the examination area as she discreetly wraps the curtain around the examination bed, allowing me to start the familiar dance, taking off my top and bra and perching on the edge of the bed, feet dangling down in front as I sit and wait for her. She approaches and stands there appraising my lopsided chest and mastectomy scar.

I instantly fight the impulse to cross my arms in front, covering to hide my embarrassment that is the flat expanse of the right side of my chest, out of place next to my remaining left breast. Even though my daughter

Carla at the age of eight has now abandoned her Barbie dolls I feel like one of them, naked from the waist up with my head turned too far around, looking out across half my back.

'Wow!' she says, and I'm caught by surprise, stunned and amazed that anyone could regard that part of me as in any way attractive. 'You probably won't see it but that's really impressive and I've seen a few in my time. I've got a great surgeon there!'

She continues her examination, asking me to lie down on my back and once I'm settled smooths her right hand over the flatness of my chest, arching around in wide sweeps, testing for any telltale lumps and then moves over to my left breast, pressing down and palpitating with the tips of her fingers, moving purposefully in a circular motion around the area of my breast to complete her examination, exclaiming, 'That's all very good.'

I get dressed, breathing a sigh of relief that I've passed yet another test and sweep out from behind the curtain to resume my seat.

'What we do in radiation therapy is irradiate the mastectomy site. It only takes a couple of minutes but we need to make sure we get the right area, so today we're going to line you up and map you. What we do is mark lines over you with a texta. In terms of the radiation treatment itself, it's painless but the most important thing to remember is you must lie absolutely still.

'Now through the course of treatment you're likely to get burnt on your chest so we'll introduce you to a skin care nurse and if you start having skin problems make sure you go and see her and she'll give you some cream to put on. We're also irradiating your collarbone as this is the most likely site for breast cancer spread but that just means you'll have an extra radiation dose each time. The main side effect from all of this is tiredness and some patients are more affected than others. So you need to get as much rest as possible. The other thing is you shouldn't be lifting heavy objects so tell your husband it's his turn to do the vacuuming! Now do you have any questions?'

'No,' I respond. After all the treatment I've had up until now I'm happy to just get on with it. After all, it's not as if I'm in any position to argue.

'Okay, I'll take you back to the cubicles and you can get changed and then we can start mapping.'

***

Back at the cubicles, Caroline hands me a white robe, and waits outside while I change. I check myself in the floor-length mirror and am instantly hit by a wave of nausea, a mixture of anxiety and embarrassment as I see its obvious under the thin hospital robe that I'm deformed and oddly lopsided as I realise I'm going to have to walk around publically for the first time, without a bra and without my soft, pillow-like prosthesis that is held in the right cup. I stand there and try to adjust my short blonde wig, anxiously checking it sits symmetrically on my bald head in a vain attempt to ensure that that part of me, at least, looks normal. When I emerge, bra, prosthesis and top in hand, Caroline picks up one of the shopping baskets from a pile and I plonk my things inside and we walk down the corridor, shopping basket in hand, back to the treatment room.

We enter the fluoro-lit, frigid radiation therapy room and to my astonishment, there are two people already there – clearly hospital staff from their uniforms: a middle-aged, balding man and a younger mousey-haired female. I hadn't expected anyone else would be in the room and certainly didn't expect there to be a man. Rather than departing, the man approaches me and introduces himself as Brett and the young woman as Emma.

Without any further preamble or explanation Brett instructs me to take off my hospital gown and shoes and to come over to the treatment bed. I look around and see that Caroline has disappeared and realise there isn't a discreet change area, only a single visitor's chair. I know I've turned bright red, instantly embarrassed and quickly try to fathom what I'm supposed to do – strip in front of him? And clearly that's what he means so I turn my back, reaching over to drape my robe over the chair to buy some time while I work out what to do, only to hear Brett say, in a slightly impatient tone, 'Come on. Look, here's a sheet you can put over yourself. Come on over and lie down on the bed.'

I take the green hospital sheet he's thrust at me and, holding it across my front, walk over to the humming machine to lie on my back on the bed, smoothing the sheet down over my chest, when Brett reaches across and quickly, without even a superfluous request, flips the sheet down to cruelly expose me, to my utter shame.

Clearly unaware or unconcerned he continues, 'Now we're going to put a special pillow under your head. Here, place your legs over this leg rest. How are your feet? Now could you please put your arms above your head? We're going to move your hips over, okay? Now, Jennifer, you need to stay floppy. It's when patients try to move themselves we have problems and it takes longer. So just lie there and let us do the work.'

They manoeuvre to position me, handling my body and twisting me into a strange contortion, slightly rolled onto my left side, with my head uncomfortably tilted over so I can only see across to my left, ending up with my arms positioned above like a ballerina.

'We're now going to take the air out of the pillow so it forms a mould,' I hear, but can no longer observe from this angle what they're doing and suddenly the air escapes from the pillow and my head and arms rapidly sink down.

Then, before I can work out what's going on I hear Brett, announcing more distantly from the other side of the room, 'We like to work in the dark!'

All the lights suddenly turn off. There's an eerie glow and a couple of spotlights instantly illuminate my chest. A whirring sound, and I feel the bed being raised, like a car being hoisted up in a mechanics workshop. Next the mechanics return and lean over me to peer under the bonnet.

'So are you going to start with the horizontal?' I hear Emma ask Brett and the next thing I know they then start to draw all over my chest with permanent textas. Diligently they proceed to mark a variety of dotted lines in red, blue and purple that extend horizontally across my chest to under my right arm. Heads down, both of them work above me as they focus, maniacally scribbling on my chest, now drawing down my middle, marking more lines and joining up the dots so the area outlined is like a large oddly shaped rectangle spanning the expanse of my right chest.

'Please try to do your best to keep the marks. We know in summer it's hard, but when you have a shower just pat the lines dry, use lots of talcum powder and when you come in don't wear any deodorant on the right side as it messes up the scan,' I'm instructed. 'We're now going to place plastic coated wires across your chest so we can scan you.'

I have no idea what they're referring to, lying there in a suspended state, increasingly feeling like a piece of meat, inanimate and without consequence.

Brett and Emma tape wires around my chest, following the texta marked lines and then just as suddenly walk out, leaving me there, pinned and lying on the bed raised under spotlights, in the dark, like some modern day sacrificial offering.

Suddenly and without warning, the solid grey arm of the machine jumps into action with a mechanical burst of sound. The arm inexorably moves, arcing around me, suddenly coming into view, its blunt end rapidly closing in on my face. I try to duck as it looms, pinned down in the cushion, my head and arms trapped. I grimace, closing my eyes, ready for the certain impact and wincing at the anticipated pain when, suddenly, the arm stops, its blunt end centimetres from my face.

A chunking noise, and I assume the scan is being done. I lie there, terrified, no problems remaining still, petrified, as I listen to the strange alien sounds, my eyes steadfastly closed, acutely aware I'm being zapped from close range. Then after what seems minutes the overhead fluorescent lights flicker on, and I realise someone has walked back into the room -- Emma – and she approaches, only to draw a couple more lines on me and then unexpectedly, announces I'm done, and it's over. A whirring sound and the bed is lowered. She helps me up, and I sit there, unsteadily, trying to recover from the ordeal.

When I finally stand she cheerily says, 'Well, I'll see you again next week!'

I shakily walk back to the visitor's chair to put on my robe and shoes. The nurse who escorted me on the tour less than an hour before, though seemingly a lifetime ago, appears as if by magic at the entrance to the treatment room and gently walks me back to the cubicles to get dressed. When I take off my robe I see a multitude of lines, some covered with tape, like I'm some sort of map. Laughably, there's even an asterisk, a radiologist's version of X marks the spot at the intersection of two lines in the middle of my chest. A couple of blue lines disconcertingly extend all the way up to my Adam's apple, and other red lines are clearly visible above the collar of my T-shirt. I emerge from the cubicle and the nurse helps me stow my robe in a pigeon hole she's conveniently marked with my name and asks, 'Would you like me to rub out the lines above your collar?'

'Yes, please,' I say, relieved and as she works to remove them, I plot how quickly I can run out of this place and back underground to the safety of my car, a private place where I can dissolve into tears.

*** 

Monday morning and I'm back to begin my six weeks of daily radiation treatment. I'm nervous. A bloody great machine nuking me from close range is not my idea of fun in the run up to Christmas. Brett stands at the edge of the waiting room and calls my name and walks me to the cubicles. After I've changed, he accompanies me along the corridor to the treatment room.

'What are the men being treated for and why don't they have any shoes or pants on?' I ask as we pass yet another elderly man, shuffling along the corridor in a robe, carrying a shopping basket full of clothes.

'Most of the men are being treated for prostate cancer,' he replies distantly. 'All right, could you have a seat here and I'll call you when we're ready.'

I plonk down in the visitor's chair in the corridor outside and deposit my shopping basket containing my clothes next to me and then dig into my handbag to bring out a wad of blank Christmas cards. This year, I've set myself the task of writing to the multitude of friends and family who've supported me through the ordeal of being diagnosed with cancer at a comparatively young age and then dealing with various forms of treatment that so far have lasted six months, happy I can put the waiting time to good use. I hear the muffled sound of a high mosquito-like buzz and a few minutes later an elderly man shuffles out from the treatment room carrying his shopping basket, turning to continue down the corridor.

'Okay, Jen, come on in,' says Brett.

I walk past the control room and into the treatment room.

'Have a seat on the chair over there,' he says, 'while we just get the bed set up for you.'

Emma places a red foam block at one end of the treatment bed and then walks over to shelves on the wall and selects a cream pillow mould, strategically placing it at the other end of the bed.

'Okay, we're ready. You can take off your gown and shoes.'

I self-consciously walk over to the bed naked from the waist up, lying down on my back and place my head in the mould, my legs over the triangular red block and rest my feet in the footrest at the end.

'Your arms should just fit up into the mould,' instructs Brett.

I lift them above my head and insert them into the appropriate places as the bed is raised and I rise up under the bright fluorescence of the overhead lights.

'So do you have a busy day ahead?' I ask.

Brett responds in a clipped voice, 'Oh yes, every day here is busy ...'

Emma plonks her clipboard down on top of my upper legs, saying, 'On the X axis we have ...'

I realise I'm not supposed to talk. I lie there and conclude no one here would notice if I lived or died. I'm just another one shuffling in to be irradiated. If I didn't come back someone else would quickly take my place.

Brett and Emma, having completed their warm up sequence, suddenly depart, turning off the overhead fluorescent lights as they go, retreating to the control room and leave me there, in the dark, red laser lines running across my chest, in a room filled by eerie green light. The overhead lights flicker back on heralding them as they walk in to continue a conversation over me that consists almost entirely of numbers, like a launch sequence.

Emma says, 'Now part of the treatment over the six weeks will include the use of this mat.' She holds up a square grey mat, half the width of my chest.

'This is going to act like extra skin.'

'What's the reason for that?'

'The beam normally concentrates below the skin so this mat acts like an extra layer of skin and draws the beam higher up. It means, unfortunately, you're going to be really burnt.'

'That's nothing,' I respond, smiling. 'I did burnt when I was fifteen. I can do burnt again.'

She places the mat on the right side of my chest. It's surprisingly heavy, like a lead weight and then before I know it, the lights flicker off again. I lie there, in the darkened room, terrified if I move a vital part of me will be nuked, forever. Then, without warning a loud buzzing sound starts that goes for twenty seconds and then just as suddenly, it stops.

The lights coming on announce Emma's return as she walks in and stands next to me, picking up a remote control and moves the scanner head around. It arcs over my head like the moon in orbit, transitioning from its secret position on the right, outside my limited field of vision, to suddenly come into view. Then, when I think it's going to continue its inexorable path, crushing my head under its weight, it stops on my left, a few centimetres away from my turned head, and I regard it in its inanimate and frozen state.

There's a sudden sound of mechanical, rapid clicking and an array of metal plates within the blunt end of the scanner head move, baring its teeth, leaving a gap within the snarly mouth the same shape as the texta marks on my chest. Emma then leaves me again, turning the lights off as she goes. Within seconds there's another intense twenty second buzzing while I try to hold my breath, willing myself to not move a muscle in case I get fried; then shallowly breathing when I realise I can't hold on any longer; and then, just as suddenly as the buzzing started, it stops.

Emma comes back in, in the darkness, and reaches over to remove the mat and then arcs the scanner back over again, this time in the opposite direction, to abruptly stop, this time its snarling mouth positioned directly above my body, poised and ready to beam its invisible rays directly down at me, like a ray gun. This round, the buzzing is short, a five second blast and the lights flicker quickly on and Emma walks back in, announcing I'm finished. The bed is lowered and I sit up, swivelling myself off as she helps me to unsteadily stand and stumble over to the visitor's chair to put on my robe and shoes and haltingly proceed back up the corridor, like some mad woman escapee from an asylum, in her dressing gown, wig askew, desperately searching for the twelve items or less check-out.

\*\*\*

I'm told the lady to ask for in the David Jones lingerie department is Bev. Time to trade in my soft, pillow-like bra insert for a proper prosthesis. I can't wait. It means that our long-planned-for family holiday in Queensland to celebrate the end of my treatment for breast cancer is in sight. I can already see myself lazing around the pool on a banana-lounge, cocktail, complete with small decorative umbrella, in hand. Time to get organised and get a proper prosthesis, one I can swim in. So I ring up and make the appointment, but the thought of going to David Jones for a replacement boob is, at the very least, disconcerting, especially when I thought their range only extended from home wares to fashion. At least it's not as strange as what I've been imagining: a shop, dimly lit and creepy, where you go to get an artificial body part fitted. I see myself, self-consciously skulking in, drawn to look up and there, above me, hanging from the ceiling, is a garish array of prostheses, different sized artificial legs and arms, all dangling from hooks. I duck as I walk underneath, drawn to venture further in, confronted by having to search through different boxes, each containing particular body parts, in the vain attempt to find the right sized boob.

The lingerie department at David Jones is full of women, all intent on the modern day version of game sport, the hunt for elusive Christmas presents. Riffling through racks of bras and undies, tracking down the right style and size, there's a crowd already there, and it's only eleven o'clock. A sizable number are genteelly jostling around the sales counter in an attempt to get the attention of the few, already harried sales assistants. There's hubbub and busyness I wasn't quite expecting.

I approach the counter and ask the youngish attendant for Bev. An older, matronly women dressed in the trademark David Jones black, emerges from behind a display rack that's incongruously filled with bright orange polka dot bras and G-strings. I introduce myself, explaining I'm here for my appointment.

'Oh yes,' she announces loudly, seemingly to the assembled throng of women waiting anxiously to pay at the counter. 'I'm not sure why I seem to be the lady that everyone comes to see for breast prostheses ... even though I am happy to help you people.'

Knocked for six by the comment, I've never been in the category of 'you people' before and I'm instantly tempted to run. Instead, Bev turns and briskly walks off and I trail behind as she proceeds in the direction of the changing rooms. She ushers me into a free cubicle and follows me in, closing the door behind us and stands there, arms crossed in front of her ample bosom, watching as I self-consciously remove my top and bra.

She critically appraises my chest, then brusquely announces, 'Okay, you look like you're a five.'

Hardly qualified to offer an opinion I venture, 'Well, if that's what you think.'

Her attitude then changes, becoming less annoyed as she asks compassionately, 'So how long have you got to go with your treatment? You're looking very red.'

The flat expanse of skin where my breast used to be is now the colour of a lobster, the radiation site clearly marked out as an irregular rectangle. Even my back is bright red for some strange reason that I'm yet to figure out.

'Only three more weeks!' I beam. 'We're going on holiday so I thought I'd better come and get a proper bra insert so I can go swimming.'

'I'll go and get the prosthesis and I'll also see if I can find a nice bra without underwire for you.' She disappears from the changing room and I stand there waiting, feeling exposed, desperately hoping none of the Christmas shoppers impatiently waiting outside don't incorrectly interpret Bev's exit as an invitation to come barging in.

There's a discreet knock and I tentatively open the door to have Bev march back in, a white bra dangling over her left arm with a medium sized white box in hand. With a flurry she opens the lid to display a wide pyramid shaped silicone object covered in a beige cotton cloth that's the shape of a breast. She places it in my hand and it's surprisingly heavy with a wobbly, slightly gelatinous feel, and I then realise why I've heard these things unattractively called 'chicken fillets'. She helps me put on the bra and then quickly inserts the fillet into the vacant cup and I stand there appraising myself in the mirror.

'Yes, that's the right size, I thought it would be,' she says, hands on hips, in a rather self-satisfied way. 'I'll leave you to get dressed. Just come out to the counter when you're ready.' She departs, fillet and box in hand from whence she came.

Emerging from the changing room, I wander out to find her back at the cash register amongst the other sales ladies who are trying to serve ten or so jostling women.

'Now you know if you've had surgery more than six months ago you're actually able to wear a stuck-on prosthesis but you may as well see how you go with this one,' she announces, loudly, for everyone to hear. 'Keep the docket because you can claim it on the government scheme.'

I feel my face go the colour of my burnt chest, feeling the stares of the assembled women, who I'm sure, have all turned to look at me.

'At night put the prosthesis into the box. It's shaped like a cradle so it will retain its shape,' continues Bev. 'Will that be on your David Jones card?'

I pray for the ground to open up and swallow me whole as I thrust my credit card at her, willing her to complete the transaction quickly so I can get out of there.

Finally she hands the card back to me and bellows, 'The scheme has only come in recently. It will allow you to claim a maximum of two prostheses so it's good when you can get something back, isn't it?'

She places the box in a David Jones bag and hands it over the counter to me. I reach over to grab it and restrain myself from bolting, prosthesis in hand from Bev and the assembled, mostly middle-aged throng of women who are anatomically complete and happily able to shop unselfconsciously for the most intimate of apparel, blissfully unaware of how normal and lucky they are.

I head back to the train station to retreat home. When the train finally arrives, I collapse into a seat, and sit there willing the train to quickly depart from Flinders Street and then realise I'd better remind myself to take the David Jones bag with me when I get off. Given my advanced state of chemo brain I know it's possible I could forget. I've heard all types of things are left on trains. The last thing I'd want to do is have to front up to the railways Lost Property Department and explain how I came to lose my boob on the train.

***

I wander down the corridor to sit outside Caroline Parkinson's room ready for my next consultation. Caroline happily pops her head out of her office and calls me in. Today she's dressed in a peasant shirt and looks more like a refugee from the sixties than the medical expert on whom my life depends. As I sit down I spot the new calendar on her wall.

'You've got my pin up girl there!' I say, pointing 'I've decided anyone who can come through breast cancer, chemotherapy and all that and still get up there and wear those gold hot pants must be doing something right.'

'Yes, my Kris Kringle. I love those gold hot pants … on Kylie, not on me! So how are you going? The results look good and you're now, what, two thirds of the way through? So well and truly on the home stretch! Can I have a look at you?'

As I take off my top and bra she winces as she sees the burn on my collarbone.

'Ooh. That's starting to look really quite nasty. I'm worried the skin might break. Is it sore?'

I nod. 'I knocked it with my engagement ring the other night and my husband almost had to scrape me off the ceiling'

'Ahh, and the rest of your chest is looking quite pink.'

'So why am I burnt on my back?'

'That's not us! It's the radiation passing through your body when the beam is above you. That's the exit point.'

*Note to myself: if I'm ever asked, I'll decline to participate in the next nuclear war.*

'I'm noticing the soreness most when I try to go to sleep at night. But the biggest problem is the seat belt rubbing on it so I've concocted a small pillow using a face washer and I've started putting that under the belt when I drive.'

'I'll get you to go down to see the skin care nurse. I'm quite worried about your collarbone but the good news is, since the Bali bombings, very good work's been done on treating burns. We used to try to keep them dry but it's exactly the opposite now. We keep them moist and the skin really heals much better. The nurse can give you some gel to use and a dressing for it. So if there's nothing more you want to ask, you can get dressed and I'll walk you down to the skin care nurse and we'll see if we can some help with that burn.'

We walk downstairs and Caroline leads me into the office of the skin care nurse saying, 'Natalie, would you mind seeing Jennifer? She's got a really burnt chest and I'm not sure I like the look of her collarbone.' Smiling, she turns to me and says as she departs, 'Natalie will look after you, and I'll see you again next week.' She leaves me with the surly Natalie who seems none too pleased with the interruption.

I stand there in the middle of the small treatment room and unbutton my shirt to reveal my collarbone. Natalie approaches and inspects, then walks over to a cupboard and reaches in to retrieve a white tube, wad of packaged bandages and a roll of skin-coloured tape.

Handing them over to me she says, 'These should do the trick. Now just tape the bandage over the burnt area after you've applied the gel. Do you want me to put all these things into a bag?'

'No, that's fine, I'll just put them into my handbag.' I stuff them in, anxious to leave and retreat home. I'll apply the dressing later. All I want to do is have a lie down and hopefully grab a couple of hours of much needed sleep.

***

I'm woken by the sensation of sweat plopping from my forehead onto the pillow. Lovely! I lie there and think it must be great for David, sleeping with a boobless, barren, burnt and bald wife. To top it all off chemo has abruptly pushed me into early menopause with the added bonus of rampant hot flushes. I struggle up, and wander into the shower, standing there under the lukewarm water, hoping it washes away the feelings of hopelessness at the prospect that cancer, my newly found lifelong friend, will inexorably come back and claim me, all the long treatment futile, a hoax and cruel game played out to merely distract me, the end result already a given.

I try to push the nagging thoughts away, knowing they won't do me any good. I quickly mop myself dry and find the wad of packages the skin care nurse gave me and get on with applying the hopefully soothing gel to the angry, red blistered area that is my collarbone. I pick up a pack and laugh out loud when I open it and see the size of the bandage which is large enough to cover half my chest, thinking I can now add partially mummified to my list of personal attributes.

I position the bandage on top of my collarbone and critically inspect to find any unburnt skin I can attach the tape to, and roll the tape out in a long strip, fastening it to my back and extending it over my right shoulder, across the bandage and down to just under my armpit. Great! Nothing like having to front up to Christmas dinner with a bandage that looks more like a sanitary napkin stuck to your collarbone. I crash down as the wave of disgust hits, like I'm on a rollercoaster as I regard my ravaged body: no eyebrows, two eyelashes on my right eye, three on my left and no lower lashes at all. Even in the wig I look decidedly moth eaten, and now I can add the extra dimension of burnt, with the prospect of having to wear a sanitary napkin on my collarbone.

I dissolve in tears yet again, and stand there, staring at myself in the steamed mirror with a mixture of loathing and abject sadness. Oh God, what have I become? Then, out of the corner of my eye, I notice something. I move closer to the mirror and reach to quickly pick up a towel and start frantically rubbing the mirror, my face hard up close to squint. Is it? Could it be? I tentatively put my right hand up to my head and gently feel, not wanting to hope but peering intently. Oh my God! It's true! I can't believe it! There's something there! There, on my head, fluff! The very first, joyous signs of life. Hair! It's coming back!

*** 

There's no better way to celebrate the resurrection of my hair than go shopping for a new dress. Buoyed with newly found confidence, I head off to my favourite dress shop in the hope I might find something I can wear on Christmas day.

'Well, hello. Every time I see you, you look different!' says the shop assistant warmly as she recognises me.

I wander around, pushing my way through the racks of summer fashions trying to find something with a high neckline that will cover my heavily bandaged collarbone. Seeing I'm making no progress the assistant professionally intervenes and pulls out a blue patterned business shirt, holding it up to show me.

'No, I'm looking for something more casual – I'm not working at present,' I haltingly respond.

'So you're on Christmas holidays?' she prompts, with pregnant pause. The last thing I want to do is confide in a shop assistant, but somehow I'm drawn to say more.

'I've been off sick for seven months, though I'm finishing treatment next week and then I'll be back to work.'

She regards me, the unspoken question hanging ...

'I'm being treated for breast cancer,' I say to fill the void, suddenly fighting back tears, surprised at myself for being so emotional given I'm talking to someone I hardly know.

'Well ...' she offers, beaming with a kind, comforting voice. 'You're looking at an ovarian cancer survivor, just on seven years now.'

'Really?' I say, completely surprised.

'Yes. Diagnosed when I was just twenty-nine years old. It took them a long time to find out what it was. The tumour was huge, like I was seven months pregnant. So I'm a good news story!'

'Yes you are!' I beam back. 'It's so good to meet someone who's a success. The press only ever report bad stories so it's hard, given that, to get it all in perspective.'

'You'd be surprised at the number of women who're treated for breast cancer. I know, because they come in here and ask for something with a high neckline, then I know.'

We talk for a while before I excuse myself, saying I better get home and attempt to make dinner. And as I walk out, I realise she's given me something worth so much more than just a new dress.

\*\*\*

Mum comes bustling into the house, ready, excited and anxious to drive me to hospital, hopefully for the very last time. All smiles, she gives me a huge kiss and I know she's just as emotional as me even though she's trying to hide it. I'm pleased she's come, at the very least to give David some respite given he did all the work taking me to the chemo sessions. Even so, standing there in the hallway as I get ready, Mum looks out of place and somewhat phased – the enormity of it all clearly evident on her face.

***

I stride up to my pigeon hole, pull out my robe, pick up a shopping basket and head into an empty cubicle, the treatment veteran I am. Mum and I then walk down the long corridor to the treatment room and I leave her in a visitor's chair in the corridor when I hear Brett call my name out for my last zapping.

I walk into the room and find Brett and Emma wearing red antlers on their heads and even though I'm feeling really very sore, their Christmas spirit is infectious and I breathe a sigh of relief that I've survived a mastectomy, chemotherapy and radiation therapy intact. No throwing up, no skin falling off, no cramping, no seizing, no really bad infections , no high temperature, no diarrhoea, no lymphoedema and, most important of all, so far, no sign of cancer recurrence.

'Sorry, but the lines have completely faded,' I apologise.

'Oh, we don't have to worry about that anymore. The target area we're aiming for is pretty well delineated by the burn!' says Brett, the red antlers on his head diminishing any remaining air of authority.

I lie down on the bed, hopefully for the last time. They go through the ritual: the countdown sequence, the lights switching off and the mosquito buzz sounds. The scanner head arcs over to blast me a second time, then the final arc back and last five second burst and, all of a sudden, it's over.

The lights flicker back on and the bed is lowered and I wobble back over to the visitor's chair to put on my robe and shoes and then bend down to hunt in my bag for the two boxes of chocolates I brought to give Brett and Emma. Hardly enough thanks for people who may have well and truly saved my life.

They each give me a cuddle and say genuinely, 'You've been a pleasure to work with but we never want to see you again!'

I turn and quickly walk out of the treatment room, not wanting to spoil the goodbye by crying, and stagger back up the passageway to collect Mum. I know I'm beaming and Mum links arms with me, giving my arm a big squeeze and we walk together slowly along the crowded corridor back towards the cubicles. Halfway along, I suddenly stop, and stand, staring. Mum stops too, looking over at me with an instantly worried expression, trying to work out what's happened as I stand there, smiling broadly, looking over at a noticeboard on the wall that's filled with pictures of cats and dogs. I stand there, in the middle of the corridor oblivious to the people jostling past, enjoying the moment. Suddenly Brett appears, attempting to walk around us as he heads back to his office. He stops, looking over at me and I point, turning to impishly smile at him.

He looks over at the notice board and then back at me, saying earnestly as he gets the gist, 'No! No really! They're our pets! Really they are.'

I laugh out loud, deliriously happy. Mum holds my hand, not getting the joke and we continue on, I get changed and then finally leaving it all behind us, we walk out together into the warm summer sunshine as Mum gives my hand another big squeeze and I know all my Christmases have come at once.

# Anam Cara

*Jenny England*

'Geoffrey!'

Within minutes that oh-so-familiar face with aging, puffy but gorgeous blue eyes and a slightly balding head appeared at the bedroom door.

'What?' he sighed.

*Where has our youth gone?* I pondered … then began, 'I need that book,' pointing to a dusty green one on the top shelf of my bookcase. 'Can you fetch it? I just got comfortable,' I continued, patting the soft pillow carefully propped under my right arm taking the pressure off my sore arm and shoulder.

Geoff carefully examined the row of books on the shelf and calmly reached up and pulled the only green one out.

'You mean this one – *Anam Cara: Spiritual Wisdom from the Celtic World?'* he said.

'Yep, that's the one.'

I leaned forward to reach for it but stopped abruptly when the sharp stabbing pain from my armpit became too much to bear. *No more painkillers for another two hours,* I thought despondently as I sat back on the pillow. *I am not sure they are working anyway.*

Geoff placed the book beside me on the bed, then disappeared.

I settled back down between the pillows on the bed, taking care not to disturb the drain hanging down from under my arm into a bag beside the bed – a constant reminder of the traumatic and mutilating cancer surgery merely a few days earlier.

I picked my treasured book up tenderly with my good hand and flipped through the well-worn pages in search of some comforting words.

Page 35:

> An anam cara in the Celtic world was a soul friend ... with your anam cara you could share your innermost self, your mind and your heart. This art of belonging awakened and fostered a deep and special relationship.

Imprisoned as I was by my pain and exhaustion, at least it gave me time to reflect on my life, but reality regularly interrupted.

'Geoffrey!'

'What now?' he called from the living room.

'I need to pee,' I called back, recognising my desperate need for some assistance. It arrived serenely and promptly.

I cautiously rolled off the side of the bed, taking care not to dislodge the drain as Geoff cleared a path to the bathroom.

'If you hold the drain, I think I can just manage,' I said as I attempted to remove my pajama pants with my left hand while precariously straddling the loo. I tried hard to ignore the razor-sharp pains and my tight shoulder. Geoff silently obliged.

'This wasn't exactly what we had in mind for our best

years together was it?' I commented in the midst of the ordeal.

'Well, at least we *are* together,' came the thoughtful reply.

I agreed.

After ten minutes or so of bathroom maneuvering and brisk hand washing I made my way back to the bed. I sighed and then continued the search for more comforting words in my favorite book.

Page 84:

> A renewal, a complete transformation of your life can come through attention to your senses ... the senses are bridges to the world. Through attunement to your senses you will never become an exile in your life.

'Geoffrey!' I called out for the umpteenth time.

'Now what! I suppose you want something to eat?'

'No, I just need a cuddle.'

# Lessons from Jack Dancer

*Elspeth Findlay*

Breasts have everything. They can be fascinating, ephemeral, taboo, delicious, essential, ugly, beautiful and redundant all in one lifetime.

My breasts are small and firm, their skin is milky and they are crowned with rosy pink nipples which seem to have a life of their own. For instance, they point in slightly different directions. I have not yet decided if that is because they have been perverted by the pressure of cloth and elastic or if they simply have different interests!

Sometimes, according to hormonal variations, my breasts droop slightly. I guess they're getting over looking perky and feel they can start to relax at their age. Generally, though, they are the sort of breasts I would have chosen if I'd had to purchase a pair rather than inherit them. But in spite of their virtues, I have seldom celebrated or even appreciated them and in truth, I have taken them for granted!

Recently, however, I have learned that nothing about life should be taken for granted. I have had the proverbial wakeup call, and it has come from within, from my own body. My breasts have transformed my life!

My left breast has been assaulted. Its soft outer swell and the inside of my upper left arm, once so sweetly sensitive, now respond to my touching with a blunt, muted feel as if shrouded in layers of coarse hessian. It is as if part of my own body is hiding – from me, from its own hands, from any handling whatsoever! It all but ignores my ministrations, my gentle cleaning and the ever so tentative massage to soften the new scars. There is only a crude abbreviated message from the damaged nerves that signify the essentials: *That's pressure, that's cold, that's sharp, that's ... something ...*

In this visceral world there's been a disaster, a holocaust. The gentle skin, the fatty tissue, the reliable muscle, the nerves which are their messengers, have all been tortured and traumatised. So now they hide, because the memory of the surgeon's scalpel is still fresh and the cells remember, even though I do not. I had to leave them in someone else's hands. I floated passively somewhere in a dark void, a place where even taking breath was unnecessary, while my flesh was very carefully dissected.

How could this have happened? How could I have been picked up like a rag doll in a tornado, and summarily dumped naked and vulnerable onto a stainless steel slab? Where now are my cherished strength and autonomy? Where now my independence and fortitude? I thought at my age I had wrangled my share of challenging characters; but I had not reckoned with Jack Dancer! This one so clever, who lives always inside and waits for the moment of weakness; waits to strike when the genetic script can be played out in a mind-body matrix weakened at last by the relentless exigencies of a life. The irony is that I had been warned, that I knew many of the Dancer's victims and I had seen them succumb and sometimes seen them die – one of them had been very close to me ...

By the time she reached her forties my mother was either in crisis management or absent exhaustion. She must have known about her cancer for some time; perhaps it played the part of catalyst because she was, at last, attempting to shed the pathetic passivity of a '50s housewife and claim back some territory for herself – her beloved bush home and her right to live independently of my father's disdain and savage moodiness. Inevitably, he had lost interest in her and the properties he inherited and absented himself from our lives to pursue younger women and the urban lifestyle he really enjoyed. It hurt her deeply, but it left her free to become herself. She deserted the kitchen for horseback and started to work in the landscape she loved, learning on the job from the men she had cooked for. She hoped desperately that she might keep the creditors at bay long enough to rehabilitate the land, the business and the birthright of her children.

But she left her run too late.

By the time I finished school and came home for good, the cancer had insinuated itself and she was miserably ill. She could no longer drag herself onto a horse, let alone muster the stamina to direct station work. There came a time when she could barely eat and she shuffled from bed to toilet like a painful scarecrow, but she seldom asked for help and never let go of the hope that resurrection might be possible. Somehow, burdened with generations of stoicism and reserve, she was unable to clearly articulate her predicament, unable to make us understand that she might be about to leave for good. I did not know how to behave or what I should do. Utterly undone by adolescence already, I could not believe that my mother would really abandon me. I was in full-blown denial, oscillating between desolation and absurd resentful anger.

Mum had to fly away for therapy several times that year but finally she disappeared into a city hospital where we children were not allowed to follow. I remember the August day when my brother put down the receiver and we heard that she was dead and in some way I felt dead as well. For a long time, whenever I woke from the respite of sleep, it was only to realise that I would never see her again.

I do see her though, because I am so like her. It's almost as if the more I declared I would not make my mother's mistakes, the more I have. Like her, I grew up in the bush and love it absolutely. I was a barefoot tomboy child, happiest among the animals and plants that I regarded as my community and like her; I was devastated when I was forced to leave it. Perhaps as a consequence of my somewhat solitary childhood, I never really learned to be comfortable in the society of people. I writhed through my school years, miserable at the confinement and struggling to manage the petty aggression of others. Similarly, Mother had been reluctant to go to social affairs and was usually eager to leave them, but we were always forced to wait while my 'charming' and gregarious father had had his fill. We learnt patience, we learnt how to dissemble and hide our angst, but we did not learn that denying our authenticity might be a kind of dying.

In the bush I developed skills that would always be invaluable – to be strong, to be invisible, to be quiet and the difference between panic and survival. In the fracture of my family I learnt to hide my internal world and manage my own despair, because the others were also under siege and dramas were unacceptable. At Mum's funeral I managed with self-absorbed rage. I was an angry seventeen-year-old rebelliously flaunting an inappropriate mini and I barely spoke – I had no time for pious gatherings and people who cared too late. I had grown into a young woman sure only of her power to endure and survive, but desperately sad and lonely. I was pretending to be the Lone Ranger.

The Lone Ranger got pretty well shot up in the years that followed. I fell out of the comfortable middle class and met people who were also damaged and desperate and sometimes brutal. I learned slowly (too slowly), that self-medicating and/or toxic relationships would not make me whole and that self-pity and denial would only keep me stuck.I was lucky that some people were caring or foolish enough to help me in spite of myself! My long-suffering grandmother, a woman of great compassion and morality, was always there to patch me up and somehow she cared about me regardless of how crass or stupid my behaviour. A good-hearted boyfriend introduced me to Buddhism and in time I began to salvage some integrity. I began to work in caring roles, trying to give something back and finally I became a nurse. I had come a long way, but I had not yet understood the whole script, the big picture – I did not see the link between my mother's mistakes and my own.

My mother was a journalist when she was married, but on her death certificate her vocation is recorded as 'home duties'. She was a skilful writer and an eloquent reader who consumed literature compulsively.

But she had very little time for her own literary expression. She was extruded into the role of housewife because she could not resist the deceptive safety of convention and because she was mesmerised by the almost irresistible promise of 'happy ever after'. I learned and understood the danger of the wedding noose, but I still did not understand how important an authentic life might be.

Caring and nurturing are beautiful when they are spontaneous and especially when they are reciprocal, but my mother had no-one to care for her and she kept no inviolable time or place to nurture herself. She did not realise that in order to survive she must insist on time for reflection and make time to write and dream, away from the demands of others. She did not understand that for those who are creative, caring is manifest in their works, their transformative gifts of insight and beauty.

In the Gnostic gospel of St Thomas, Jesus is quoted as saying, 'If you bring forth what is within you it will save you. If you do not bring it forth, what you do not have within you will kill you.' I think that my mother died of several broken hearts and one of them was creative. She could not express what was within her and so her inspiration finally turned to empty frustration and despair and ultimately became her nemesis.

Unconsciously I had become stuck in the same toxic paradigm. My early attempts at rebellion had ended in failure. I was not as brave and strong as I thought and I took cover in the acceptable role of carer, unconsciously acting out the internalised script of my mother and generations of women in my family and others: 'Abandon yourself, abandon your passion, your role as a worthy woman is carer!' An ancient recipe and a deadly one! I also carried in me the deep fear of poverty and humiliation that goes with losing a home and I could not resist the juggernaut of consumerism that pervades our lives.

I had inherited the protestant work ethic and secretly craved the faux security that money buys. So I worked in a worthy job fulfilling the role of carer; the useful, the conformist, the taken for granted good girl trying to manage the endless neediness of those who cannot help themselves.

I lived in a constant welter of worry and tiredness, internalising the stress of others as well as my own and it pervaded my home as well as my working life. I limited my creativity to writing academic essays for nursing studies and ignored my muse. It was a rare moment when I felt inspired to write poetry or prose. Like my mother, I read the works of others and listened to them on radio obsessively, but I procrastinated when it came to my own expression. In truth I was conspiring against myself, preparing a fertile ground for the familial tendency they call cancer to express itself. I too was nurturing my nemesis!

When I heard the words, 'I'm so sorry, you've got two lumps in your left breast, you have breast cancer', I was barely surprised; there was no alarm or rage, just an internal recognition.

My doctor was concerned. 'You seem very calm!' she said.

'At my age my mother was dead,' I replied benignly. 'I'm living on borrowed time anyway.' It was as if my mother's destiny was my own, as if that made it acceptable. Actually, I was also well on the way to losing my faith in life, tacitly giving the nod to death. Driving home I thought about the arc of my life and the times I had been tempted to end it. Now all I had to do was nothing and that death wish could be fulfilled; I was being given a legitimate solution to an unfulfilled life. It was time to make a decision.

I think that's when my mother really reappeared, when a vague memory of her began to morph into someone with a presence, someone insistently in my mind. I had lost a lot of her, perhaps out of sadness, perhaps out of anger, but the cancer brought her back to my consciousness. She was not the only one. As others found out that I had cancer they appeared from unexpected directions and gave me flowers, vegetables, medicine, advice and other gifts – they let me know that they cared in ways I had not dreamed of.

My partner showed how beautiful a man he really is, a stalwart hero who loves me enough to put his own life on hold and listen to my panic and sadness, drive me everywhere, dress my wounds, act as supporter and advocate and a buffer against the world. I was able to resign from the petty tyranny of inappropriate work and think carefully about what it would take to really honour and enjoy the life I had been given.

I would have to write, to disregard the dire warnings about starvation and useless self-indulgence echoing in my old thought patterns and focus instead on fulfilment, on a better and more heartfelt way to give something more than just dogged service. I wanted to give something inspirational for myself and for others. I had decided to do more than just survive.

I started immediately. Before I had to have surgery I managed to attend a writers' workshop and it was uncanny to find that the main exercise was to write about our mothers!

I wrote: *And she appeared!*

Even in the deepest greyness of her life, my mother was extraordinarily noble and strong, but in the story that came to me, she was also mysterious and powerful. She appeared, no longer in the conventional dress of a housewife, but in the living, chimerical garb of an elemental, and she had something for me. Her gift was a creative kernel of inspiration drawn from the natural arc itself. A gift from one artist to another – I was enchanted!

In the months that followed we travelled miles, to appointments with surgeons and specialists and physiotherapists. I spent time in hospital and learnt what it is like to be a patient, a valuable insight never gained from all those nursing years. I was helpless and befuddled and sore, but I had time and my laptop and I could write!

I am still writing and it is not easy, but it is like voyaging – always a challenge, always something new emerging from the sea inside. Slowly my flesh is regaining its senses and my muse clamours for attention. I have the gift my mother gave me, a reawakening and another chance. I have come back to my authentic life!

# Know When to Run

*Yvonne Fein*

It took a malignant tumour on my left breast to convince me that my forty-a-day habit was probably not an optimal lifestyle choice.

Mind you, I had kicked the habit before.

During both my pregnancies, some moral whisperer got the password to my conscience and kept murmuring, 'Hey, your kid's getting the habit. In utero. That can't be right.' So I stopped. For nine months. *Twice.*

By the time I came to, after the operation – lumpectomy, excision of lymph nodes, tubes to the left of me, concerned relatives to the right of me – I'd endured two days of nicotine deprivation. When visiting hours were finally over, I attracted the attention of a passing nurse.

'Dying for a smoke,' I gasped weakly.

'I could probably scare one up. Might take a while.'

I gave her a martyr's smile. I could wait.

When she finally returned, she slipped me the contraband and kept her voice low. 'You'll need to go to the visitors' lounge with those,' she advised.

You see, children, back in the day, there were still dedicated areas for smoking in hospitals.

'Those?' I looked down at my palm.

'I got you two, love. Don't smoke them all at once, now.'

I trundled along to the smoking den, wheeling my drip with one hand and clutching my hoard in the other. They were Turf cigarettes, a brand no longer available over the counter. Their tar content was so high, you could have laid down a length of freeway using a single pack.

Botting a light from another patient I sucked deeply on heaven's edge. The rush was instant and magnificent. The paper burned and crackled around the precious tobacco, eating up the bitter smoky infusion far too fast. I lit the second off the butt of the first. My world narrowed till there was nothing but the inhale followed by the slow, lazy exhale through my nostrils and the sharp, smouldering acridity coiling and twisting into my eyes.

Returning to my room I started to feel strange. Not the strange of the nicotine high but the one where saliva starts gathering and no matter how much you swallow, it keeps coming. I started to jog, keeping a tight grip on my intravenous meals-on-wheels. I reached my bathroom just in time to deposit a huge gush of mystery fluid – I'd eaten and drunk nothing for the last forty-eight hours – into the merciful white of the porcelain. And I kept retching and heaving until every single morsel I'd been fed since the day of my weaning was gone.

After that, I never smoked, never *wanted*, another cigarette. I didn't even have the dream – you know the one all ex-smokers dream where they've taken a puff and wake up in a pool of self-recriminatory sweat.

That was it for me and it's been nearly twenty years.

***

BC (Before Cancer) I was something of an emotional asphyxiator: if I experienced intense feelings, I'd push them down till I'd suffocated them. I didn't realise I was simultaneously cutting off my own vital oxygen.

That said, I'd dealt resolutely with chemo, hair loss, the disappearance of my periods, the curtailing of my ability to work, the questions of my children and the fears of my parents.

I was doing great.

Then it was time for radiotherapy.

Dr FeelBad's assistant's first words were, 'You're late!'

I'd arrived fifteen minutes past the hour, red-faced and distressed. All the emotions I'd been happily asphyxiating over the last thirty-six years were roiling inside me, looking for a reason to erupt. She gave me one.

'Do you think I wanted to be late? I got lost, the car park's like Christmas Eve at Chaddy and this rabbit-warren of a building badly needs signage. I wish I'd been on time. I wish I didn't have to be here at all, but I do. I've got cancer and you're talking to me as though I'm a school-kid late for Maths. Is there anything else you'd like to say?'

An alien had invaded my brain and body. I welcomed this furious stranger as though he were a lover I'd been waiting all my life to meet.

The first words Dr FeelBad himself said to me were, 'Your hair. That's odd. It shouldn't have grown back that fast.' Then he demanded the results of my blood test. I told him my oncologist had not taken any blood. He insisted she had.

'You just forgot because of your stress levels.' It was the only time he smiled.

Adrenaline still pumping from my encounter with his assistant I replied, 'I may have lost half a breast but my memory's still good. Ring my doctor and we'll sort it out.'

He hesitated, my certainty giving him pause. Eventually he discovered I had not indeed had the infamous blood test but he never apologised. And this set the tone for future encounters.

He was a great, strapping man who wore his health rudely. He also often wore a safari suit to work. A trekker, a hiker, a great outdoorsman, for some reason he would regale me with his exploits through Africa or across the Annapurnas. Struggling just to walk to the park, I felt inadequate and depleted by his tales.

Since diagnosis, I had been working closely with an extraordinary psychologist who specialised in hypnotherapy. She taught me how to focus on the radiation rays so they healed me from the inside and kept the radiation burn to a minimum on the outside. This seemed to vex the good doctor no end.

'You should have more intense reddening on your skin,' he told me more than once.

One night, provoked beyond sleeping by his latest expression of malevolence, I wrote him a letter. I know I covered at least two pages but the only words I actually remember are:

> *I honestly believe you do God's work, but you're a bully. People consult you in their most extreme vulnerability and instead of reassuring them you intimidate and torment them. All your expertise cannot compensate for the fear and antipathy you elicit.*

Once my treatment was over he wanted to see me twice yearly for check-ups. In refusing, I realised that cancer had taught me even more than how to kick my addictions and verbalise my feelings. Vital though these things were, somewhere along the way, like the gambler in the Kenny Rogers' song, I had also learned when to walk away and when to run. This would help me keep my head and my heart.

It would keep me alive.

# Poised

*Marietta Elliott-Kleerkoper*


a state of unknowing
not a wilful turning away–

the yes and the no hovering
like the needle

on a fine set of scales –
forever seeking equilibrium

the cat in Schrödinger's box
alive and dead

the results of my bone scan
positive and negative

sooner or later I will receive
information that will destroy

this balance–for the moment I remain
poised in ignorance

# Breast Cancer Yarn

*Helen Armstrong*

**January 2010**

I'm on record as saying that I hate mammograms. When I turned forty-five I did choose, however, to take advantage of the full extent of free mammogram monitoring.

'It is only momentary discomfort,' I was told. 'Mild, transitory.'

I was unprepared for the feeling of skin being ripped from the flesh and the corner of the plate digging into my armpit lymph nodes. After repeating this over several years, I cried uncle. Or aunt, as the case may be.

**January 2005**

I told my GP, 'When the obviously male inventor of the mammogram machines deigns to put his gonads on the glass plates and have them crushed for my amusement, then I'll consider it. Until then – no more mammograms for me.'

I took comfort in a family history that was blessedly cancer-free. Well, mostly. But there are always isolated cases, aren't there?

Five years passed. My husband began to be increasingly concerned as I kept ignoring the BreastScreen reminder notices. At his insistence, I asked my doctor about alternative monitoring methods.

'What about ultrasound?' I asked her.

My GP explained that ultrasound examination is not a substitute for mammograms, merely an adjunct. Taken together, they better visualise the nature of anything of concern that may have been found. Alone, ultrasound examination of the breast is of limited help. She emphasised that mammograms should not be painful. Also there are new machines out now and newer techniques. She convinced me to give mammograms another go.

**29 January 2010**

I was apprehensive but, in fact, I breezed through the process. Glory be, at last a mammogram that did not leave me with lasting pain! It was so easy, I wish I had returned sooner.

A week passed during which I told many other women that at last mammograms are easier to endure and certainly worth the peace of mind they can give you.

**5 February 2010**

I got a letter from BreastScreen:

> Following your visit to the Breast Screening Service, we would like to ask you to have some additional X-rays.

The letter reassured me that there wasn't necessarily a problem. I had to ring to confirm the appointment, which was still a week away, and again felt reassured. 'Most call-backs are just to make sure there isn't a problem,' I was told. 'Better to make sure.'

**11 February 2010**

The BreastScreen clinic at the public hospital was low-key and efficient. I was met by a woman who explained to me that they needed to repeat the mammogram on my right breast because there was a small, slightly brighter patch that they wanted a second look at. It was probably nothing but better to be sure – after all, that's what mammograms are all about. After the mammogram they would probably also do an ultrasound just to take a different kind of look. Both together would really help see what was there, if anything.

I held onto the 'if anything' and got ready to have a relaxing hour or so out of my day. After signing consent forms for the repeat mammogram and the almost-certain ultrasound, I was shown to a change room where I was told to remove my bra but leave everything else on.

I thought, *Why a change room for that?*

Like most women, I can whip my bra off without removing my outer clothing – sort of like the party trick of pulling the tablecloth out from under the crockery. It's even easier when you're only wearing light summer clothing. So I removed my bra, stuffed it into my bag and a little self-consciously entered a room with about five other women, all in similar stages of breast-sagginess. I felt the room should have been labelled over the door, 'For the fallen'. I noticed one or two women wearing cotton gowns over their skirts.

There were tea and coffee facilities so I made myself a cup of coffee and rummaged for a magazine to read.

As I glanced around the room I saw a basket containing wool in various shades, knitting needles and an assortment of partly completed knitting. The notes in the basket explained how to knit squares 'wrapped with love', so I took up one partly completed piece and began knitting. The TV was on but nobody was watching.

It's always the way with knitting – you always get interrupted. I was called for the mammogram before I had barely got halfway through the first row.

This mammogram was a bit more uncomfortable than the one two weeks earlier, but still not the agony of past painful experiences. The technician was very efficient; she only worked with my right breast and neatly sandwiched it horizontally, then vertically. I was back to the knitting within minutes, but via the change room again. I would need an ultrasound, so therefore I needed to change into a gown.

These gowns were of a soft cotton and in various pastel shades, like patchwork fabric. Against bare skin the cotton was more pleasant than the scratchy paper fabric of a disposable gown. I noticed that there were now only three women all gowned, plus a young woman who was there as companion – possibly a daughter to the quiet older woman sitting with her. Oh well, waiting times would now be shorter.

Barely into the next row, I was called for the ultrasound. Again the staff member was female. In fact, the only male I saw all day was a man who seemed lost and was asking the clinic receptionist for directions. I hoped for his sake he wasn't there for a mammogram – men can get breast cancer, but trying to do a mammogram on the very small amount of mammary tissue would be a difficult procedure.

The ultrasound operator was a doctor. Before she began she showed me the previous mammograms – from five years ago, and from two weeks earlier. There was clearly a small bright area on the new mammogram.

When she did the ultrasound, this same bright area showed up as a dark ellipse. Because she was a doctor, she was able to talk to me as she went, showing me on the screen what she was looking at.

'It looks like a cyst,' she said. 'In which case we will want to aspirate a bit of fluid from it, if it has fluid, just to make sure there's nothing of concern in there. Most of these are benign.'

She did tell me that if the fine needle was unable to draw off any liquid she would want to take a small core biopsy, rather like drilling for ice cores in the Antarctic, only in miniature. She would do it as soon as she had completed the ultrasounds on the other patients.

Feeling a bit more reassured ('it's only a cyst') I returned to the knitting and finished my coffee. I was called away (mid row again) to sign the permission forms for the biopsies.

Interrupted again. Another half row. This time I defiantly brought my knitting with me. Another woman wanted to feel my breast. Judging by the level of quiet respect shown to this newcomer, I figured she was a more senior doctor.

'I can't feel anything,' she explained to me. 'Even though I have seen the pictures and I know exactly where it is.'

*Can't be too bad then.* Back to the waiting room.

Again I was part way through a row of knitting

when I was called for the biopsy. Back to the ultrasound room, same doctor I had first seen doing the ultrasound. Another woman, obviously a nurse/technician at the very least, was also present. She chocked me up so I was lying partly on my left side, right boob uppermost but still covered.

When the doctor came back in they set up the instruments tray and uncovered my boob. I was swathed in a large green drape with a neat rectangular window exposing a few square centimetres of bare breast. I knew I would need local anaesthetic – I hate it. Anything that involves injecting a liquid volume into a part of the body that doesn't have room for it is going to sting a bit. It wasn't so bad, however. The ultrasound probe had been gelled, plastic-wrapped, then my skin was swabbed with antiseptic. The doctor injected local into the skin and then deeper into the tissues. By this stage I was not feeling the deeper injections. The nurse held the ultrasound probe in the place directed by the doctor and I was instructed to not move while the doctor carefully aimed the needle into the heart of the cyst.

I could see the doctor's face as she concentrated, but it was a bit too difficult for me to watch her and also watch the screen. She got the biopsy needle in, then attached a syringe, carefully giving sharp, quick tugs to the barrel of the syringe to aspirate from the cyst.

But no luck.

Thankfully I had already signed the permission to do the core biopsy, because everything was already set up. It made sense, especially while I was already mostly numbed for the needle biopsy. The doc apologised for the necessity and injected more local, deeper into the tissues. I felt nothing of this other than a little pushing. Then the biopsy needle – I had to be very still again. I could feel the pushing but there was no pain.

'A little click now and it could sting for a second,' she warned.

I heard the click and felt a slight, brief discomfort. I've had a liver biopsy and this was a breeze in comparison.

The doc withdrew the needle and put the tissue sample in the tube. 'I want to try for another,' she said. But then she seemed to change her mind again. 'No, we've got a trace in the fine needle biopsy, and that tissue sample as well should do.'

That was it. The nurse applied a gauze dressing to my breast for a minute, applying pressure. She applied steristrips over the very small hole, now barely oozing. She stuck a dressing to my breast; it looked like the same stuff the 'no bra' adhesive breast supports are made from. The nurse then wrapped up a small disposable ice pack and told me to hold it firmly to my breast for twenty minutes.

Although I was not in any pain, I was rather shaky when I got up off the table. My spirits were okay, as I was still feeling confident in the doctor's unofficial opinion that this was probably a cyst. But the experience of having a needle pushed deep into my breast to sample a piece of tissue from near the chest wall had been more of a shock than I had considered. No matter how gently done, it is still a bodily insult that you should never discount.

Back in the waiting room, one woman had already had her biopsy, same experience as me, while the other two waited their turns. I made myself another cup of coffee, somewhat horrified at my shaky hands almost spilling the coffee granules. The teaspoon made the tremor visible. I was glad my back hid the coffee cup and my shakes from the other women. I didn't want them to feel alarmed.

As I held the tiny ice pack in place we began to chat. The woman with the daughter didn't seem too inclined to talk, other than wanting reassurance that the biopsy process was fairly painless and gently handled. The woman who had already been biopsied was called and told she could go. Meanwhile the other woman and I chatted until she was called in for her biopsy. While she was gone the nurse came in with sandwiches and orange juice. Lunch. The quiet woman's daughter was also given sandwiches, which was very kind of them.

After about half an hour my chatty friend returned. Lunch had been left for her also and I think she was relieved to have something to distract her. I was still clutching the little ice pack to my breast and realised I'd held it in place for forty minutes – plenty long enough. I took it off, tucked it into my bag and took up my knitting.

The quiet woman was called out and soon returned, dressed ready to go. The nurse brought her an envelope to take to her doctor. Then my chatty friend was called to see the doctor, then soon returned, dressed to leave.

I was the only one left. The nurse called me in and told me what was to happen from here.

'The pathology results are being rushed through for everyone. They're really good about that here. We'll have a narrow window tomorrow at about lunchtime when our surgeon will be here to give you the results. Or if you would prefer, we can fax the results through to your doctor and you can get the results closer to home.'

I'd already decided to do that. After four days in a row having to be away from home, driving into the city and enduring the heat, I wanted a quieter day. They made sure I had already made the appointment for the next day, then told me to go get my clothes back on. I had a sheet of instructions to read on wound care including a strict injunction to not get the wound wet until next morning. So no swim after all.

I felt a bit conspicuous being the last one there, but it wasn't for long. I was on my way soon enough. I got home at about 3.00 pm feeling a bit drained by the experience and by the heat. I'd gone in for a quick repeat mammogram and after four hours I'd also had an ultrasound and two biopsies.

**12 February 2010**

Next morning I removed the dressing. The day was even hotter; I was glad to not be driving through the heat back to the clinic. By late morning I was down at the beach enjoying a gentle swim and sunbake. The water was warm, the sand scorching. I sat leaning against a smooth rock and let the sun warm my breasts. The events of the previous day seemed too bizarre and distant from the peace of the beach.

A cool change blew through mid-afternoon when I headed out to see my doctor. She was running late; it was almost 5.00 pm when she saw me. She took her time, opened my envelope and put the mammogram pictures and the ultrasound images up on the light box. She showed me the cyst image on the ultrasound.

'The report says it's clear and defined, but here the margins are a bit blurred,' she commented. She seemed to be stalling, going through all the information meticulously. Finally she said to me, 'I'm sorry to have to tell you, but they have found cancer. The pathology is definite. It will require more examination, you understand, but provisionally they've described it as Stage 1 or 2. You have invasive ductal carcinoma.'

Her previous dithering had forewarned me, so I wasn't upset. I was surprised, however, since I knew I was very low risk. I've grown up convinced that I would never get cancer. *We don't get cancer in my family* was the belief. This is despite my having a brother with prostate cancer, a niece with breast cancer and a great aunt who is perhaps the oldest mastectomy patient on record, at almost 100. Somehow I managed to dismiss these as anomalous. Plus I had been told that because of my own auto-immune condition, I was extremely unlikely to ever get cancer.

The GP seemed to need to reassure me, but I felt okay. I sent a text message to my husband, who immediately rang me. Meanwhile the doctor was calling a surgeon to set up an urgent appointment for me. I left a few minutes later, waving cheerfully to the receptionist.

Outside I sent a text message to my kids and a couple of friends. With poor reception it took about fifteen minutes. All this time my mind was going furiously. *I have cancer. Me. Not possible.* But it's definitely for sure. No doubts. But it's small. Ten millimetres. That's thumbnail sized.

It will be okay, they will just take out the lump, maybe a couple of lymph nodes and it will all be contained and gone. A bit of radiation treatment to make sure, and it will be done with.

The message I sent said:

> I have a dx of Stage 1/2 invasive ductal carcinoma, I see the surgeon on Tuesday. I'm OK though.

### 16 February 2010

Surgeon appointment, this time a very anxious husband was with me. He seemed torn between his own panic and a misplaced need to reassure me. But somehow, perhaps because of the gradual process I had been through already, I was feeling centred. Part of me was a little jittery at the knowledge that inside my breast was a turncoat set of cells gone rogue at some stage in the past and only now discovered due to the latest medical sleuth technology. I wanted it gone. Whatever it took.

The surgeon was a surprise. Young, female. I knew she had been my friend's surgeon. My friend's prognosis had not been good, and she is still with us and now completely well. So I should be fine. I was in good hands.

We sat opposite the surgeon. 'I'm sorry to have to tell you that this is invasive ductal carcinoma,' the surgeon said. 'But it is small. As I said to you last Thursday, I couldn't even feel it.'

Wait – last Thursday? So she must have been the much-respected doctor who felt me up while I was more focused on knitting. I really had not recognised her. The powers of self-distraction …

I asked, 'If it is so small, how can you know if it is

invasive?' My family had been asking the same question since the diagnosis.

'The sample we took spanned the margin,' the surgeon explained. 'So we got a sample of the tumour, a sample of normal tissue and in between we could see that the tumour has already broken out of the duct.'

She went on to explain the process as gently and swiftly as she could. 'We'll bring you in for day surgery and remove the tumour. It's about the size of an olive. We'll also take a chunk of healthy tissue so we can make sure we get clear margins. It will all go to pathology so we can know what type it is and whether it is hormone-receptive or not. What we find will determine what happens from there. Radiation certainly. Chemo too, but only if we have ongoing concerns. We won't get those results for a week or more. But we will get lymph node results, at least preliminary ones, while you're on the table.'

She went on to describe the sentinel node biopsy procedure. 'The day you come in for your surgery, you will be first sent to Nuclear Medicine. They will ultrasound the tumour again, and under ultrasound they will insert a hook wire directly into the heart of the tumour. They will also inject a radioactive tracer. It's the same stuff used in bone scans. Then we find which lymph nodes are first in line from the tumour. It may be one lymph node, but usually it's two or three. They will be marked and they are the ones we remove at the same time as the lump. They go to Pathology; we wait while you're under anaesthetic, then if pathology tells us they're cancer-free, we close up. If Pathology is concerned, we remove all the lymph nodes in that armpit. Pathology study everything in more detail and we get a thorough report in a couple of weeks' time.' She also told me she would be injecting blue dye into the tumour and using that to confirm which lymph nodes were 'hot'. 'So don't worry if when you wake up, your breast looks a bit blue,' she smiled.

I was told about the cancer care team, a multidisciplinary team who each put in their oar and come up with a best plan for each patient. I signed paperwork for the surgery, paperwork for the cancer team, more paperwork than I could follow.

We were given a choice – wait for a public bed, perhaps a month, or go private and get it over with faster. I wanted it gone, so we went for the private option. I was booked in for the following week. We left, me feeling a sense of determination pushing me onwards.

**17–21 February 2010**
Over the next few days we told more people. I felt uncomfortable with their reactions. People kept looking at me sidelong, clearly concerned.

Finally my husband said, 'You're too calm. I'm worried – you should be screaming, crying, yelling, "Why me?" but this calm, almost happy coping is something that scares me. I don't want you to come crashing down. You can let go – I'm here for you.'

And he was – but I was okay. I had a job to do, I had tasks to get underway. Immediately after my diagnosis on my way back to the car, I bought some cheap knitting needles and a couple of balls of yarn. I began to knit squares with the same fierce determination.

I did take time to think. In my life were a lot of unfinished projects. While I was almost certainly going to be all right, this was a wake-up call. It was time to re-evaluate the direction of my life. Current projects – my writing. A play I had just become involved in. My son's home schooling – he has high-functioning autism and needs support. I would need to cut back, but I could use my energy more efficiently.

I was not prepared for the reactions of my friends. Some who I knew had been through this were open and supportive in practical ways. One long-term friend surprised me when she said, 'I went through this ten years ago.' She had never said a word, had denied me the opportunity to support her. I felt angry with her, but of course we all cope in different ways and she is a private person.

Male friends were supportive but almost intrusive at times. One said, 'I will miss seeing you in that beautiful low-cut red dress.'

I replied, 'Stop worrying. Nothing will stop me from wearing that dress.'

He said, 'Knowing you, you've probably got all your crying over and done with.'

'Not at all,' I told him. 'I haven't cried at all. What would be the point?'

A friend in the US was distraught. She choked up and was unable to speak for some time. 'If you, such a strong person, can get this, what hope is there for the rest of us?'

'It happens to anyone, strong or not,' I told her. 'I will get through this. Perhaps I am a reminder to have your check-ups. I'm eating my anti-mammogram words now.'

I went through my days with adrenaline driving me on.

**26 February 2010**

The day of surgery came and we set off early. At the hospital everything ran in organised sequence. After announcing myself in the foyer, I was sent to Nuclear Medicine for the hook wire and isotope injection.

I'd been through the biopsy, so this should be no worse. However, this time I met the first male health professional in my cancer journey. He was quiet and gentle, but it threw me a little. This man was going to touch my breast. I was lying on my back in a darkened room and, for the first time, feeling apprehensive.

The radiologist, also male, entered the darkened room and explained what to expect – I'd heard it before. The local. The wire to be inserted, a guide for the surgeon, to make sure she took out the cancer primarily in one neat piece and didn't have to take out too much healthy tissue in trying to find it. The isotope injection directly into the tumour.

It went smoothly. My tumour was above the nipple, quite high on my chest but against the chest wall inside. A long way in. The wire end was taped to my breast and, still gowned, I was sent to wait for half an hour. I tried to read a magazine but the words made no sense in my head, so I knitted. Soon I was called again, to a different room. The technician led me to a seat in front of a large machine and I had to sit there, arm up, and wait while my body was 'read'. Then the radiologist was back and removed my gown. He drew on my breast and armpit with a felt pen. Two crosses in my armpit showed that two sentinel nodes had been identified. I looked at my body – the felt pen marked where I was going to be scarred.

We were finished in Nuclear Medicine, so I dressed and we were sent back downstairs to wait, near the lobby. A lot of things had happened but I still felt I was waiting to be admitted – when was I going to become a hospital patient? It felt like a practice run, not yet real. And yet it was.

A nurse took me to a private room so we could talk. More history was taken and she talked to me about what to expect. She gave me a cushion, donated by Zonta, a world-wide organisation working to advance the status of women. This cushion was a beautiful pale blue satin in a crescent, designed to pad the wound area under my arm and breast to reduce discomfort after surgery. The nurse also gave me what seemed to be a showbag, with some brightly coloured information packs in it. Plenty of useful reading to keep me going.

It was now after lunch and I was still in the waiting room.

Finally they came for me. 'You need to get into a gown quickly. They are ready for you in theatre.'

No time to think, no time to sit in the bed and stew about it. I barely had time to go to the toilet first. I think I spent about five minutes sitting on the bed after I had the gown on before it was time to get onto a trolley and be taken to theatre. That was when I had to wait – I spent more time waiting on the trolley before surgery, than in the bed.

I was finally feeling scared. However, I kept telling myself that I was in good hands, and that this had to be done. I had an invasive tumour in my breast and it had to be removed. I wanted to know urgently how bad it was. And the only way to know was to get it all cut out and have it examined in minute detail. My nerves were showing in irritability. When the anaesthetist came to get me, he had his nose outside his mask. I told him that his nose had better be inside his mask during the surgery. I don't think he liked me saying that, but it would be my body having to deal with the infection in the tissues if his strep got loose.

I knew instantly when I came round that it was over. Before I even opened my eyes I reached for my right armpit with my left hand to feel for the level of surgery. Wonderful – only a small bandage, and no sign of lymph node clearance! That meant the sentinel nodes had been negative on examination.

Eyes still closed, I mentally assessed myself. I felt fine but shaky due to the greater body insult. I was undoubtedly more in shock than after the needle biopsy, but that was understandable. I'd had the equivalent of being stabbed in the chest. The surgeon told me afterwards that she had removed the tumour as best she could, then examined it before sending it to Pathology. That was when she realised she had misjudged, and possibly not taken enough on one side. It had been a little bigger than expected. So while the lymph nodes were being examined, the surgeon went back in and removed more of my breast to make sure she got clear margins. It was probably a good thing she did -- the Pathology eventually showed that the first sample was within a millimetre of the tumour. The second sample was completely clear, so she had got the margins clear after all, but without that second sample, we would not have been so sure.

All I had to show for it all was two small patches of dressing. One on the top of my breast, the other in my armpit. My top was moderately low cut but didn't show anything of the bandage.

**27 February 2010**
I was not supposed to drive for twenty-four hours after the anaesthetic and I had a meeting I wanted to attend. Undoubtedly it was foolish and a certain amount of denial of frailty, but I went to my meeting. My husband drove me, and stayed nearby. I was still feeling a bit shaky but I was glad to be there to do my job. I think I was focusing on being useful. We left early, I went home to bed, to rest. For a breast that had had a golf-ball-sized piece removed, it sure didn't seem any smaller. If anything, it was bigger.

**28 February 2010**
By the next day the bruising was much more obvious. The bruise now stained beyond the area of the dressing; my boob looked like Gorbachev's birthmarked head. We began calling it Frankenboob, and christened the bruise Robert, a veritable King of Bruises. Robert the Bruise. My cup was definitely running over, as my increasingly swollen breast declined to fit into any of my usual bras. I was wearing a maternity singlet top I had bought just before surgery. This was soft, comfortable and had supporting cups. I lived in that top, wearing various shirts as overwear.

**1 March 2010**
I began to feel mildly feverish a day later and I was put on

a course of antibiotics. Perhaps it was the extra bruising caused by the second tissue removal that was the reason. Infection is fairly common.

Superhuman me was, however, still trying to pack in as much productivity as possible. I had a dental appointment coming up towards the end of the week, but things went badly awry when I had a vomiting attack from the antibiotics. My son says I have Black Knight Syndrome, a reference to *Monty Python and the Holy Grail.* ''Tis but a scratch,' says the Black Knight, blood gushing from the stump of a severed arm.

After the infection began to subside, things quietened down. People asked me what operation I'd had. I said, 'Two weeks ago I had cancer. I don't any more.'

I felt confident. The lymph nodes were negative. I had a great surgeon.

### 11 March 2010

When I returned for the detailed pathology results, the news was still good. The lymph nodes were confirmed as negative, the tumour had been a slow-growing type, and it had been hormone-receptive. That meant I would be taking medication to block the tumour's access to my body's hormones. But wait a minute – what tumour? My cancer was now in the pathology lab, not in my body.

The surgeon explained that it almost certainly was all in the pathology lab, but there was always a faint chance that a cell or two may have got loose. It was time to talk about making sure that all the cancer had been eradicated. Time to use both belts and braces.

Radiation treatment would be needed. I was concerned about what this would do to me, but I was told it was chemo that was tough to endure and made hair fall out.

'A lot of people keep working through radiation treatment,' I was told.

My husband was going to take time off work for my radiation treatment. There were plenty of people willing to drive me to the hospital for my daily treatment, but he insisted it was his job only. There was no rush for radiation; I had six months or more, they said. They would let me know when a slot became available for me.

I considered my timetable for the year. What could I drop? What did I want to persevere with?

My writing. I wanted to do more, not less. Well, writing is something I could do while resting.

What about the play? I was increasingly concerned there were more problems than I felt I should have to deal with. When the production was cancelled I was relieved.

**March–April 2010**
My skin healed up. There was a hard lump at the surgery site and I looked like my boob had been scooped out with a melon baller. The scar was curved, parallel to the upper edge of my nipple but several centimetres higher. It looked ugly. And it was still sore.

**6 May 2010**
My initial radiotherapy appointment at the Cancer Centre. This was when I was measured, photographed, tattooed. Two black pinpoints – a brief sting for each. One was between my breasts, the other under my arm. I was guided around, shown the ropes. A practice run.

The Cancer Centre staff became my next focus. The Cancer Centre was going to seem like a second home, the staff like family. I accepted a place on the STARS project, a large database following breast cancer patients. Blood tests and someone else deciding if I would begin medication at the same time as radiation, or after. In my case – after.

**24 May 2010–30 June 2010**
My radiation treatment began. Each day we rose early, drove to the Cancer Centre and went through our morning routine. I always wore a bra support singlet top under my clothes, instead of a bra. I would arrive at the centre, walk in, greet the receptionist, make a cup of coffee then find the knitting basket. While I waited and knitted, I talked to other people waiting there. Women, men, patients, partners and friends of patients. We talked, we compared notes and as treatment progressed, we passed on burn management tips.

When my name was called, I went in to the waiting room for my particular 'machine'. I had my own pigeonhole in which to store my own gown. It was a blue paper gown, the same one for most of the treatment. I was supposed to go into a change room, remove my upper clothing and put on the gown. I soon found what worked best for me – I would stay out in the waiting room, strip down to the singlet top (which was perfectly respectable), slip the straps demurely off my shoulder, then wrap the gown around me. As the staff got to know my method, I often did not have time to even do this much. If they had a five minute window, they generally knew I could be in and out faster than most. It was good for me – less waiting. More time to get back to my son and his schooling.

Once I was called in to the treatment room, I was asked to lie on the bed of the machine. I peeled down my singlet top, then covered myself back up with my gown for as long as I could. There was always a cold draught in that room and it was not just modesty that kept me wanting to stay covered. Various trays and boards were added on to support my arms. I had to lie in exactly the same position each time. The pinpoint tattoos on my skin helped them line the machine up exactly the same each day. They would draw on me with felt pen which often showed above my clothing later. My right arm was up and over my head; my left arm was supported at the side near my waist. I must have looked like a topless, recumbent highland dancer.

I would lie there in the semi-dark while I watched the red laser beams line up across the walls and ceiling, and form roadmaps on my body. Then the lights would come on, a bell would chime and the staff would leave. I was alone with the machine. It would buzz for seventeen seconds and I counted each one. Then the staff were back, re-checking alignments. Then another seventeen seconds of buzzing solitude.

On the ceiling was a beautiful trompe l'oiel mural of a tropical scene with butterflies. It was designed to look as if you were peering up through the window of a conservatory, onto a tropical scene – palm fronds visible. And butterflies. I counted eleven butterflies in total.

There was another butterfly garden mural on the wall but I couldn't see that one except as I was quickly dressing afterwards. All I had to do afterwards was pull up my singlet top, fold up my gown and pull on my shirt. No more need to use a dressing room.

I didn't have to go every day. Just most days. Every second week I would get a day off, to give the roster a chance to squeeze in an extra person, or machine maintenance.

After my first day of treatment, I was immensely drained. I just wanted to curl up and sleep somewhere. My treatment also meant I was not home to get my son started on schoolwork each morning, so a teacher at his correspondence school would telephone him every morning and talk him through his routine. Some days we brought him with us, then after my treatment we continued on to the school so he could meet with teachers for more intense tuition. Often my husband stayed in the classroom while I crawled back to the car to catnap.

I had been warned my skin would begin to break down, and I should use moisturiser. But there was to be nothing on my skin before treatment. I carried my creams and my aloe vera leaf with me and began to apply it after each treatment. No oils, they said, but allowed Sorbolene. But I developed folliculitis and I think the Sorbolene was part of the problem for me. So I made up a spray which was mostly purified water with a fraction of a drop of tea-tree oil in it. I would spray that on my skin after each treatment and the folliculitis stopped getting worse.

The skin breakdown was inevitable. I did not have too much difficulty with it – another woman I spoke to had problems for weeks with blistering and the need for dressings. She was the one who advised putting the stuff (cream, gel, or even honey as she was using) on the dressings, and not directly onto the skin. To apply stuff to the skin when it is damaged and delicate risks rubbing off layers. I greatly valued that advice.

My skin began to blister two weeks before the end of treatment. The treatment team were vigilant and immediately after their daily work sent me to the nurse who applied gauze dressings. I had other heavier cotton pads to hold it in place – nothing could be stuck to the skin. The trouble was, the plain gauze was still too rough and when I showered that night the dressings came off and took skin with it. Next day a different nurse applied wet gel dressings and gave me more of the same to apply.

I would open the packet to reveal a square of net, impregnated with something like glycerine. To this I applied a swirl of clear gel and spread it evenly to cover the dressing. Then I applied the dressing to each blistered and burned area. The gel glued the dressings on with no need for the adhesive tape, which was not possible given the skin breakdown over a large area. At first I only had a small blistered area, but soon my breast was papered with these jelly dressings, looking a little like shingles on a roof. Over the top of these I applied gauze, and over that I applied cotton wool padding. I tucked it all inside my singlet top, using the top to hold it in place. I had a brainwave – I got some disposable stick-on nursing pads and sanitary pads and stuck them inside my clothing. I had permanent dressing padding now. When I gently rinsed off the dressings it was difficult to tell what was dried gel coming off and what was sloughing skin. Some areas became raw and bled.

The burns of course continued to worsen for another week after radiation finished. The day after my last treatment, I also had to start the anti-hormone pills – Arimidex, in my case. I started them on 1 July 2010. I'd been apprehensive but didn't notice much change.

I found Arimidex caused problems with sex – a vaginal tightness that started almost immediately after I began them. Eventually the doctors switched me to Tamoxifen. Tamoxifen works by a different metabolic pathway, so its effects are a little different. But the important thing is, like Arimidex, it prevents any possible tumour cells from feeding on hormones.

I told the drug company about the problem. They were surprised, said they had no prior record of this specific problem but did find reports of women complaining of painful intercourse. I am lucky – I am in a stable long-term active relationship. How many women going through this do not have the opportunity to find out? Perhaps they think, *After all I've been through, I have to accept some negative changes in my body,* and don't bother the doctor with it because, well, it's not life-threatening like the cancer.

Immediately after surgery I had an over-large bruised boob. Over time it lost the swelling and settled somewhat. But the firmness of the scar meant that the shape was more obviously odd. All swelling had gone by the time radiation treatment started at the beginning of April. By the time radiation treatment finished, the scar was softening and the affected breast seemed smaller and floppier, as if radiation had turned it into a shrinky dink. I was not happy about its shape or size, although I had to be grateful to still have some breast. I'm told that with mastectomy, the loss of cleavage is an unexpected shock when you look down and can't help but realise what has had to be done. To most observers I look unchanged by all this. They sigh with gratitude that it is all behind me now, a short, unpleasant distraction from life's usual bustle. But to me, I would look down and see how v-necked shirts would always pull to the left, the larger boob filling the top more generously. Dammit I LIKE to wear v-necks!

**10 August 2010**
I needed help with good bra fitting. At first I went to the bra department of a major store. I explained my situation as post-breast cancer surgery. They tried in vain to fit my now mismatched boobs. I was told with amazement that my DD bustline was now a C – I realised afterwards that they were only looking at the scarred breast, not the normal one, in the same way parents with twins, one handicapped, risk paying all attention to the sick twin and neglecting the healthy one.

**12 August 2010–28 August 2010**
I rang the breastcare nurse. Again. They were by now recognising my voice over the phone. They gave me a brochure for a couple of services for prosthesis fitting. I rang the nearest one and found she worked from home nearby. She was an expert – just looking at me she came very close to an accurate estimate of my real size and what I needed. Measurement only confirmed her estimate. I still needed DD. But yes, my shrunken boob was closer to a C. Normal bra fitting was going to always be difficult now.

She ordered what I needed and two weeks later I was back, husband in tow. I brought some of my secret weapons in the fight against the hassles of cancer treatment. My favourite low-cut top; my trusty black maternity singlet; and a sexy underwired nightie, which I had actually worn to bed for weeks immediately after surgery, to help support a very tender boob. Surgical and sexy. She was intrigued. How we each have to manage is very different, depending on where the scar is, but this could help others with a scar in a similar high position.

I left with two new bras and a new swimsuit, each with a mesh lining to hold my new silicone prosthesis. My partial prosthesis looks more like a chicken fillet and I did say, 'Maybe I'm being silly, I didn't really lose that much, not as much as others do,' and she hushed me.

'You know your body, and have a right to feel comfortable with your body. This is not silly.'

We went straight to a friend's party, the same male friend who had commented sadly that I could never wear THAT red dress again. And I wore that red dress, with my new bra and prosthesis proudly perky. He gave me a hug, a few seconds longer than perhaps necessary, and thanked me for giving him a lovely birthday present – me, restored. Hmm. Oh well, he's a bloke. Maybe it's as close as he can understand. But it did do my self-esteem a power of good.

## September 2010–November 2010

In all the changes and difficulties I had to face, I did not find any unpleasantness or hassle. Instead, it felt as if I was wrapped in comfort and support all the way. Treatment was streamlined and whatever I needed was there at hand, proffered as my need became apparent. With all the fundraising for breast cancer, let me tell you, it is paying off big time. If only the rest of the healthcare system could run as smoothly!

## December 2010

I went to file my Medicare claim for the bras and prosthesis. I made sure I had everything correct. I rang from the local pharmacy's Medicare counter. I was shocked to find the first unhelpful, nasty operator I have ever encountered in all my years of making Medicare claims. The problems began when she asked for the bra fitter's provider number.

'There isn't one,' I tried to explain. 'This is different to the usual claim. It's for a prosthesis following surgery for breast cancer.'

'How many times in the past have you had this done?' she asked.

'I've only had cancer once, and it was only one breast. What do you mean, "How many times?"' Again I tried to explain. 'I was told this needs a different type of form, a pink one, not the usual green one. I have the receipt, the account was paid in full. It should all be okay.'

'Stop telling me what is going on and let me ask the questions!' the operator snapped. 'It sounds like you've been conned. I'm sorry to say that there are too many tricksters out there. You can try to go back and get their provider number, but from what you say this person wasn't even a doctor. Who referred you?'

'The Cancer Centre,' I told her. By this stage I was angry, but at the operator because I knew this was covered; it was definitely legitimate and my kind prosthesis fitter had been most careful to do the paperwork correctly. So I tried to play the game. 'Could you tell me exactly where this has gone wrong, so I can tell the Cancer Centre? They deal with a hundreds of cancer patients a week, they need to know that their advice that they have been giving for some years is badly flawed. I'm amazed nobody has made that clear to them.' I was hoping to subtly make it clear that the Cancer Centre staff must surely know what they are doing. But no dice.

The operator spelled it out for me as if I was an idiot. 'Every service requires an item number and every service provider requires a provider number. We also need the provider number of the referring doctor. And you say you self-referred, from a brochure,' – I could hear the sniff – 'given to you by a *nurse*.' Her tone of voice was obvious – a mere nurse was never qualified to make referrals.

I thanked the operator, stupidly did not get her operator number, and hung up. Then I burst into tears.

In all I had been through in ten months – the shock of the diagnosis, the pain of the surgery and biopsies, the reaction of family and friends – I did not cry. No tears. Just got on with it. And now, for the first time, I cried. Not for the cancer, but the shame I'd been made to feel, as if I was a criminal trying to extort Medicare, as if I had requested elective surgery and faked breast cancer solely for the purpose of being able to claim for a breast prosthesis.

Two weeks later we had the chance to go to a Medicare office. I took the same paperwork and mentally steeled myself for more trouble. But the staff there were lovely, kind and processed the claim uneventfully.

## January 2011

A lot has happened since my diagnosis of breast cancer. It is now a year since my mammogram that started it all. I have made a lot of progress with my writing in that time. I completed a large knitted blanket which I donated to a needy family, and I've knitted other items which were also donated. My knitting is always with me and I have increased the challenge. I use my time better. I don't feel I'm on borrowed time, or on a time limit, but I am grateful for what I have and not wanting to waste time. I am more ready to say no to certain tasks and also I have noticed I am far less patient with those who I feel are wasting my time.

But otherwise, I am still me. And I am still here. And hope to be for some time to come.

## 26 February 2011

I went for my twelve month post-breast cancer mammogram. It hurt like hell, because it's post-surgery. But I will never miss a mammogram again.

# The Three Rules of Cancer Club

*Mark Dean*

London is expensive on Valentine's Day, more pricey than usual and you can't get a table for love. The Tube doors opened to Tash saying, 'As we are over west for this appointment, there is an Italian pizzeria I want to try.' It was then two years after her primary cancer. She was at that point twenty-seven-years-old and this, along with her mother's early passing, were the reasons why we were standing on the up escalator of Sloane Square Station that particular Tuesday evening.

February in London is cold and dark. A furthest point away from beautiful stirrings of love and beauty the date implied. The Tube was empty even though it was still rush hour. Tonight the metropolis seemed split between those that had somewhere to go and the rest who were already indoors, alone or otherwise. It was no surprise that the station was sparse and that there were even fewer people out on the bleak streets. There was just us, walking.

If you drive across London, you'll recognise where we went – the old Edwardian red brick on the corner of Chelsea Bridge Road and the Embankment, along from the Royal Hospital where the flower show is. Tash had been referred here by one of her treatment team in Sydney. He had spotted something. The genetics team at the

Royal Marsden Hospital are the best there is. Innocently we had not considered why they had persisted in trying to contact us.

'Don't worry,' Tash said. 'This will just be a quick visit. We will be out again in a minute.' After this evening I would tell her to not say things like that again.

Dr Eeles sat in a rather small room – not only small, but because this venerable building had had several masters already, each with a use more removed from the original, the room was the weirdest shape. Not the expected rectangle. Dr Eeles herself was a nice woman, thin, wiry and very Médecins Sans Frontières. We got to know her well, but this initially was not to be a pleasant meet and greet.

Sixty minutes later we left. Neither of us had spoken for forty, even when Dr Eeles enquired, 'Any questions?'

There were none. We just got up and left.

Whilst I cannot say that either of us remember the meeting with clarity – the words that Dr Eeles had said, the descriptions, the statistics and the probable outcomes – we left retaining the bleak statement that, genetically, Tash's abnormality grouped her with only sixty other family groups in the western world. Bleak words that in a few years would become the basis of our joking comment that, considering the type of cancers she could have had, she should have had, the fact that she only had secondary Breast Cancer, which is rather treatable in the larger scale of things, was a bonus really.

But tonight that evolutionary thought process was yet to come. We were walking up a very cold street in the dark London night, cocooned in a disaster that might be. Tash can be curt at the best of times, and at the worst she maintains the Bella Figura with an iron fist, but she was silent. I had no grand thoughts, I just wanted this to be a mistake, but knew already that it wasn't.

I broke our silence. 'I am not hungry.'

She replied, 'No, neither am I.'

I finished, 'Let's go home then.'

I never knew her to do this again. There are two types of people: the weak and the rest of us. The rest of us are not always strong. We fear too, but we also know that fear has its place and this was one of them. If we were a castle, our feeble defences had been truly breached; the forces to lay siege to us now camped well within sight. They had simply pushed a little and our walls had fallen. This would simply not do, no, not at all. There was no fight from us; we both understood that this could not be the way.

If this is the future we are to be given, we revealed to each other without words, then this is not how we will approach it.

We would clearly have to regroup.

\*\*\*

There are Three Rules of Cancer Club:

1. Have a party
2. Buy some shoes
3. Go on holiday.

This is how we lived, because cancer is not about death, it is about living. Live you must, when your mortality is challenged. And live we did.

Under these rules I have watched Tash twirl for hours, shoes discarded, her feet bare on dance floors, front rooms and backyards of London, Sydney and Verona.

She would dance, she would smile, she would move, twirling one hand in the air and the other piloting it's own upward spiral holding a Jack and Coke. There she would stay into the early hours, until the party would end, and home we would go, my wife whooping, punching the air in celebration of a good night out. She always looked wonderful, not glamorous in hiding, but luminescent for Now. From her head to her toes a glorious escarpment of the best you could buy. Our flat overflowed with clothes and shoes, so much that she would hide her illicit scarpe at work, sneaking the massed footwear back on nights I was out. When we finally took her home, we made sure she looked good: her best shoes, her best frock, her best as ever, her last. Always the most beautiful Bella Figura.

There was always a holiday before treatment, a *piss off* to the prescription.

The first: back home to be married.

'Don't try to arrange your wedding from the other side of the world in six weeks,' she informed our guests triumphantly as we dined at Aria embraced by the Opera house, Bridge and Harbour.

The last: to Iceland. Really, she was too sick to fly, but wanted to go, so we went anyway. From Sydney through Sicily, Verona to Paris, Mallorca, Sweden and around again, everything was always possible. My albums of photographs now digital chronicles of life once lived; bright sunsets, close poses, pictures of living as statements full of intent. Only now I see, in the back of her smile, the knowing that we could never avoid the-what-might-happen-next.

When I held her maybe, maybe she could. In those moments I would write cheques I knew I could never cash, borrowing the strength to keep ahead of her by sacrificing any of me. I did this because I loved her, I did this because I knew I could, because I wanted to. All she wanted was to lead a normal life and all I wanted to do was make sure that she could.

In the end, perhaps we lived more than that.

\*\*\*

'Quick, get a bucket.' It was almost a whisper.

I half gazed up from FHM, and then back again.

'Get a bucket quick! I am going to be sick! From the toilet, hurry.'

This is a strange thing to hear in the circumstances, especially when it jerks you away from an article on 'Boobs and Beer in Bulgaria' and makes you focus upwards to see your wife sitting resplendent on a white leather dentist type chair minus the dentist. Nothing other than her, me on a very uncomfortable plastic chair, shoehorned into the curtained cubicle and a long steel pole holding the litre and a half of diluted clear chemotherapy wired down her arm. Strange, suddenly, is not descriptive enough.

'Bucket!' she snapped through understandably clenched teeth.

I am English and she is Australian. There are cultural differences. Had the situation been reversed I am sure this gung-ho Aussie would have leapt to my aid. As it was I just sheepishly enquired, 'Do I have to?'

She growled her response and I snapped into action. This Oncology Unit was long, hi-tech and very, very hushed. I showed my wife all the intentions of immediate action, my running motion morphing into an expectant walk as soon as the curtain closed. My gait, though, belied the conflict in my mind. 'Quick! Bin! Vomit! Toilet? Where?!'

Toilet, she said, so I went out of the swing doors, into the corridor at an increasingly brisk pace, increasing with every vision of taking a vomit-stained spouse home on the Tube.

The toilet had a very small bin. Had a gerbil vomited, this bin would be overflowing.

Fuck.

Fuck ... Fuck.

I didn't want to, but had to. I soo didn't want to make a fuss, I didn't want to utter the words, I didn't even know how to say them. Umm wife-mine-vomit-maybe?

'Help!' I whimpered across the desk of the nursing station. Clearly in their eyes, the only help I needed was a stiff drink.

'What's wrong with her?' the nurse replied.

I explained in quick one syllable utterances.

'Ohh,' she said. spreading a calm around me, and then my wife, as she pulled back the curtain, handing one of those odd kidney-shaped dishes to her. The type of bowl that looks like it should be for the other end, but smaller and made from recycled paper that makes you unsure if it will contain any liquid or just soak it up, turning in to a vomit paper wheat-germ mess.

There was to be no vomit today. The nurse turned down the drip and her nausea passed leaving just the two of us engulfed in a pregnant silence that can exist between two people after a puke-bin-chemo incident such as this.

This could go on for days. I broke the silence.

'What bloody bin?'

'The one in the toilet,' she laboured in a manner that clearly indicated that I was an enormous idiot and a failure of the highest order for not knowing exactly which one she was referring to.

'The big bin?' I ventured blindly.

'Yeeeaah.'

'Oh,' I quietly ended this part of our jousting. 'You mean the big bin in the toilet that you go to, don't you?' I asked, poking the now cantankerous bear in my midst with my finely worded stick of light revenge.

'Yesssss!' I was going to get a belting in a minute; it was all in her eyes.

'The toilet that you go to,' I repeated, 'with the enormous yellow sign on the door that says Patient Toilet – Patient Use Only. For Transference of Chemotherapy Waste. That toilet, you mean ... that obviously has this big bin.'

'Oh yeah.' She started to realise. 'What, you've never been in there then?'

'Is it my arse hanging out of a hospital gown?' I replied.

We laughed.

What else could you do?

\*\*\*

We flew in to Mallorca in September then drove into the old town of Palma. It was a gloriously sunny afternoon.

Spanish hot, like the Chorizo, peppery in the light, prickly on the skin. The old town was a disaster, too many streets, too busy, too pokey, not enough signs. I swore at her directions, she criticised my driving, we laughed after a fashion and parked outside the city walls. The sun started to burn our skin. Map in hand she added some distance and I paced behind her up the cobbled hill, a walking Buckeroo, two bags balanced on either shoulder, our suitcases in either hand. Her shoulder hurt, she said; I was not surprised. 'There must be twenty magazines in your bag.' There we were, hot on holiday.

The bright sun from our carefree Mallorca set behind a working October in London. She still complained of a sore shoulder. I brought her a new bag, a proper rucksack, not a skeleton-twisting shoulder bag. But her shoulder was still sore. She is not one to complain, but is one to spend money. First one physiotherapist appointment, then another. By the fourth visit, he had bought his Porsche and she was no better.

Soon, the physio's influence was to melt away in the face of the behemoth that was to rise to claim her again. Once every three months we hold our breath. Over ten airless days we respire for each other through one combined anxiety. Many tests, many different rooms, many different machines, bleeping electronica acting as the hand of fate to our next quarter.

Together we try to skirt the inevitable conversation; soothsaying over dinner, predicating the future based on little more than runes and false confidence.

'I've had some stabbing pains in my liver again,' she confides.

I countermand with care, 'I don't think it is more cancer, dear. You said that last time and we were fine, remember?'

She will pause, shrug, then tell me that she does not know why, but she isn't so confident that we will be okay this time. I will, as I always do, put aside my fear and tell her it will be fine. This time she is scared, last time it was me. Here we are, gambling on outcomes we have no influence over. Forming our fears into armour that will be useless against a *fait accompli* delivered at the oncologist's office.

When the results are good, we exhale and start to breathe again, taking a slap on the back for surviving the unsurvivable once more. If not, then we wheeze for sixteen weeks, her treatment becoming incorporated into our normal routine. This is how Secondary Cancer lives with us.

Her first scan, an MRI on Wednesday, curtails any thoughts of a clean escape.

'The oncologist called,' she tells me that evening, delivering the most difficult of sentences, a *coup d'état* on herself. She maintains her composure. 'They've detected a narrowing of one vertebrae. This could be either osteoporosis or bone metastasis.'

The food in front of us becomes cold as we contemplate our choices: a wheelchair or a significant slip down the darker and deeper.

Thursday becomes a dead loss. We spend Friday together in the bowels of a building. Tying her gown, light blue to light blue and dark tie to dark. I make idle egg-shelled conversation as we sit uncomfortably in a corridor while she forces down a pint of white drink, comfortably coloured, and not the radioactive yellow that you'd expect for a bone scan. The weekend falls quietly beside us. The following week contains scans to the second Wednesday; CT, PET and UCA. Tests so complex that we only know them by acronym. This mirrors our life. Not living. Just an abbreviated existence.

We meet after work on Thursday, thankful for the distraction of the 9–5. The taxi silently navigates the rush hour to Harley Street. The driver reads our mood and does not converse. The oncologist's office is her domain. They have a relationship; she offers herself more to him than me. He is the *a trois* in our marriage. Without him, there would be no us and he has only eyes for her. Tonight he is a harsh lover, straight to it, translating the radiologist's report. His lips turning speculation to ugly concrete. The pain in her shoulder. It is her spine. Her T4 vertebrae. More cancer. Somewhere new.

We exited out onto the street. It was a stark November night. I was unravelling.

'I want to go home,' I told her.

She fixed me with a stare colder than the air, caring, but some things are more important. 'No', she said, 'I have booked the bar, people are expecting us, we are going out.'

Now the First Rule; we will deal with the rest tomorrow.

Tonight we are alive.

# Stepdaughter

*Joe Dolce*
*for SVH*

You are daughter
yet not daughter
the old language was stepdaughter
but there is no step between us

my hands moved
through your hair
as a girl as a woman
now you've asked me
to take it all off
before the chemicals
can do it

facing away from me
your open neck exposed
my bright scissors cut
away years falling to the floor

an electric shaver leaves
furry cap and finally
my hands full of warm lather
a whispering razor's edge
you're newborn

Stepdaughter

except for the now revealed
remnant cicatrix from childhood
when you smashed through
the car's front windscreen
before seat belts

I towel you off
hand you hand mirror
you regard yourself stoically
but still manage some laughter

now you are looking at me
with all the surrender of the world

you are daughter
yet not daughter
the old language was stepdaughter

but there is no step between us

# Treatment

*Sara McKenzie*

You are going to be honest. Starkly. There is no point putting on the rose coloured glasses that everyone wants you to. Over the past year you have been hurt more than you care to remember. The pain is palpable, real, sometimes a shout but most of the time an insipid whisper that never leaves your head, like the Wiggles' songs that your son wants played over and over again.

**INT. GP'S OFFICE - DAY**

**Dr Doctor:** It feels harmless. But I always like to get a second opinion anyway.
**You:** Okay. So you don't think anything's wrong?
**Dr Doctor:** No, that's the most harmless breast lump I have ever felt in my life.

You don't really feel relief but you force yourself to. You make an appointment with the breast surgeon believing that there is nothing wrong but you had better make sure. When you enter the building, your stomach turns and you realise that nothing will ever be the same again. There is nothing overt that tells you this and you don't know why. Is it intuition? Is it your imagination? Is it even real?

## INT. BREAST SURGEON'S OFFICE - DAY

**Dr Surgeon** is a middle-aged woman whose smile is constant and genuine. She apologises for the wait and her terribly cold hands. You see the city stretch out before you in the window behind her and feel the smog encroaching on the building.

**Dr Surgeon**: How old is your son?
**You**: Fourteen months.
**Dr Surgeon**: How beautiful. You can bring him in, you know. We don't mind at all.
**You**: Thanks.
**Dr Surgeon**: Are you still breastfeeding?
**You**: Yes.

She feels the lump. The fact that it hurts is a good sign that there is nothing wrong, she says. She tries to aspirate it to see if it is a cyst. Then she sends you for a biopsy. It is a simple procedure just to make sure but it seems fine.

**You**: If there is something wrong, what will it be?

You are hoping there are other options other than cancer. She answers you but her words are muddy and dull and don't tell you anything. You hold onto the word *fine*. You run it through your mind. This time you believe it.

**INT. MEDICAL SUITE - DAY**

**Radiologist:** It looks like just a cyst.
**You:** Oh, good.

Enter **Doctor.**

**Doctor:** Let's take the biopsy.
**You:** He said it was a cyst - can you just drain it?
**Doctor:** No. It doesn't look bad, though.

You hold onto the shock as the needle clicks your flesh and pretend you are fine. You don't want the doctor to know that the jolt upset you. He is tall, sniffly and has the 'God awful lurgy that is going around'. You try not to breathe in his spittle. He sends you off for your mammogram.

The radiologist squeezes your breasts into pancakes, stretching and pulling them between the hard plastic panels. Meat in a sandwich. You marvel at how flat your breasts have become since breastfeeding. She tells you that they are still full of tissue unlike the elderly.

You suddenly fear what will happen when you get old. She looks at the screens.

**Radiologist:** Any history of breast cancer?
**You:** No.

This is a routine question, you tell yourself. Your breast bleeds profusely on the way home. You can feel it seeping through your bra on the tram. Nothing feels right but they have all seemed to think nothing is wrong. When you get home you tell your husband it will all be fine. The look in his eyes tells you that he doesn't really believe you.

You watch as your fourteen-month-old runs and rolls on the grass, laughing. He cuddles you and kisses you and you hold him tight and smell his hair. That night, he lies close in the darkness, feeding, drawing comfort from your heartbeat. Neither he nor you know that this is one of only a few more times he will be allowed to do this.

**INT. YOUR HOUSE - MORNING**

It is the day of your results. You are heading out the door.

**Husband:** Should I come with you this afternoon?
**You:** No, there is no point taking time off work. There is nothing wrong.
**Husband:** Are you sure I shouldn't come?

**You:** Yeah. All you'll be doing is taking time off to hear her say that I am fine.

You kiss them goodbye. Confident. But there are cracks.

**INT. SURGEON'S OFFICE – DAY**

When you step into her office, you know immediately. She doesn't say anything and her smile is just as wide but there seems to be a dull look in her eyes, like someone has painted a film of grey over Van Gogh's Sunflowers. Dr Surgeon starts talking about your scan and holds it up to the window. Her words bumble and jump and you are listening intently, not wanting to miss a word and not at all because all you can think is, *Why isn't she telling me there is nothing wrong? If there is nothing wrong wouldn't she have said it as soon as I walked in?*

And then ...

**Dr Surgeon:** So, I am going to turn your life upside down a bit now.

You feel the tears spill messily down your face.

You cover your mouth.

You knew this was coming but her words stab at you anyway.

**You:** Am I going to die?
**Dr Surgeon:** No.

Dr Surgeon hands you a book called *Early Breast Cancer* and a website that she likes. She tells you to go home and absorb the information and come back for another appointment after further tests to discuss the next step. She looks genuinely sad but leaves you with the secretary anyway.

You feel there should be something more.

Isn't there more to say? Can't she take the pain and shock away? You know that she has done this many times and that the drama has worn off, that her real expertise is in the operating room and in a funny way you are shocked, resentful and thankful at the same time. You pay your fee quickly, trying to hold in the flood, trying to stay calm.

You hear the words *mammogram*, *MRI*, *ultrasound*. You know your life has changed and that every fear you ever had is living in your body now. You are sick. You have cancer. You have a husband and a son.

You feel betrayed.

You have felt this many times but this time it is your body that has betrayed you. The grief overwhelms you. It is time to say goodbye to everything that was. The future is scary, wild, quiet and sad.

**INT. HOSPITAL - DAY**

The day of your mammogram, your husband comes with you. He holds your hand in the waiting room and you try to joke about the shows on the medical TV channel. You are scared. And when they inject you with the blue fluid, they tell you that you cannot breast feed for forty-eight hours.

You didn't know this but the night before when you were nursing your baby to sleep, you closed your eyes and breathed in every moment of it, thinking that this could be your last chance to hold him in this way.

You were right.

**INT. YOUR HOUSE - DAY**

Your sister rings you every day. You can feel her choking back the tears. You know your mother cries when she is away from you. Her face is crumpled with worry, her mind filled with all the possible darkness that could ensue.

Over the next few days you cry. You worry about whether you should get a mastectomy or a lumpectomy. You want to hurry up and get the cancer cut out of you. You want a clear answer from someone, anyone, but it is all up to you.

At night your husband holds you while you cry and say that you don't want to move forward, that you can't do any of it. You can feel him breaking inside, feel his mind in despair ... He tries to stay strong for you but you know him well enough to know that he is feeling the same grief. This is like death for all of you.

You are operated on, bruised, tired. You have a CAT scan, a full body bone scan, meet your oncologist for the first time. He tells you to be real, that even though your cancer was caught early that you are young and that it is oestrogen positive and that the tumour was over two centimetres so something has to be done. As your denial starts to shred away, he strikes the final blow.

**INT. ONCOLOGIST'S OFFICE – AFTERNOON**

**Oncologist:** There is no good news at the oncologist.

Silence.

You feel stupid and small. You had hoped that cutting it out and having radiation therapy would be enough. Suddenly it is a lot more real.

People don't like your sadness, your fear.

**MONTAGE OF WELL-WISHERS:**
**Person 1, 5 and 7:** Be positive.
**Person 2:** The glass is half full.
**Person 3:** At least you have your family to help you out.
**Person 4:** Try to think positively
**Person 6:** You will be okay.

Friends disappear, some stay. People have advice; give you books on natural therapies. Apparently beetroot juice works wonders. You read about a farmer who developed a vitamin cure for cancer. *Too much phosphorus in the soil causes cancer*, he says. *The doctors are ignoring the facts*. On the internet people pedal miracles and you wonder why the medical profession exists at all. You hear countless stories of friends and family members of other people who have had cancer. They were all always worse off than you, they all battled it with a smile, they all stayed strong and so very positive and never had a down day.

You want a t-shirt that says:

> *Just because I am sad and scared*
> *does not mean that I am being*
> *negative; it does not mean that*
> *I think that I am going to die.*

You always were an atheist. This experience hasn't made you find God. You now know for certain that He doesn't exist.

You are going to be honest. You hear stories of inspiration, of strength, of lives changing for the better, of rebirths of awakenings after cancer.

You have to be honest and say what you feel.

If someone asked you if you could go back in time and change it, would you? You know many would say no, that they have found something deep inside themselves, that they have learnt so much. You feel ungrateful when you say, *Yes, I would change it; I would wish it had never happened.*

You would tell them that in every photo you look at you think about whether it was before breast cancer or after it. You would explain that your mind is filled with grief every day and that you never stop thinking about it. You would tell them that even though they cut out the cancer, there is no going back, *ever,* and that this is enough to break your heart a million times over. You would tell them that trying to be strong only makes you weaker and that you have started to learn to relent to the pain inside you and have let it find its own place to live – somewhere where you can watch it, somewhere where you can see it every day but where you don't have to visit. You would tell them that you are sad, that it hurts, that it kills you a little every time you think about the possibility of it coming back. You would tell them also, though, that even though you would make that period of your life disappear if you had a chance, that there is still a voice inside of you that holds on. It holds on because it has to. Somewhere inside you there is also a hope that tries to survive and that even though it is not a lot, it is enough to live by.

**EXT. CITY - DAY**

You walk through the buildings, your feet splashing the rain water that has soaked the pavement. You look sad, pensive. The camera pans up in a swooshing motion up to the sky, moving over the city and the river. There is a film of smog but the sun is shining on the roof tops.

# A Friendship Too Short

*Katie Flannigan*

My breath froze as I exhaled. Being heavily pregnant my body was hot, but the night was not. We shuffled uncomfortably on the unforgiving wooden benches in anticipation, like nervous athletes keen for the start of the game. I was one of thousands who spilled on to the grass of the Melbourne Cricket Ground prior to an Aussie Rules Football match.

It was winter 2005.

And it was a first.

We wore flat shoes to preserve the hallowed turf and pink plastic ponchos to support the Breast Cancer Network of Australia (BCNA). The plan was to form a giant outline of the Pink Lady logo of the BCNA and then fill her in. Like colouring in with pink human pixels. By the end she looked radiant against her grassy green background. The event was called the Field of Women.

There were fourteen thousand of us representing the number of Australian women diagnosed with breast cancer each year and a handful of men in blue ponchos to acknowledge that men do suffer from the disease as well. In Australia three thousand mothers, sisters, wives, daughters and girlfriends die every year from the disease.

We were there to raise awareness. I was there for two women: Lyn whom I knew professionally, a breast cancer survivor and the visionary who founded the BCNA; and Leanne, a past employee and good friend who was six years into remission – so not technically a survivor, not until the seven year cancer-free milestone. I remember snippets of that evening. It was both emotionally charged and busy.

Emotional because the massive scoreboard showed the results: the numbers diagnosed, the number fallen and celebrated them with photos and messages from loved ones to music. Tears and memories and broken hearts.

Busy because I took my daughter Georgia, positioning us on the edge so as not to get lost in the squash. With the recently found freedom of toddlers' legs, Georgia took every opportunity to practise her mobility, breaking ranks from beneath the ribbon fence that traced our outline. One newspaper printed an aerial photo of the Pink Lady with a tiny stray pink pixel escaping the pack closely followed by a much larger, beachballish one. It was madness to go by myself but somehow deeply important. I wasn't there for me. Had Leanne been in Melbourne she would have been there and it would have been fun and positive.

Leanne was tough. She'd moved from Western Australia to work with me and my team. She pushed me as a manager and as a friend. Assertive, fun, professional, ambitious but memorably tough.

Simon, whom she later married, called me one Friday night to tell me the news: 'Katie, Lee has just been diagnosed with breast cancer and is having surgery over the weekend and we don't know what that's going to mean. She won't be in on Monday.' Leanne was twenty-seven at the time.

At that stage Lee had worked for me as an occupational therapist for five years and in that time built her own caseload and referral base. I took over her clinic on the Monday morning and felt deceitful telling her patients, 'Lee is not in today, she's not well but will be back as soon as she's better.' I am a lousy liar, although it wasn't really a lie, but wasn't really the truth. I saw all her clients that day then rescheduled them with other therapists for follow up appointments.

There was one patient, however, who stood out that morning. I had already received a fax and a phone referral by 9am for him and now he had appeared at the clinic needing to be squeezed in to an already full schedule – the usual treatment for a VIP sportsman injured over a weekend.

Patrick Flannigan, as it turned out, was indeed a VIP suffering a sports injury but not exactly a VIP sportsman. He asked a lot of time-consuming questions, acquiesced unhappily to being rescheduled with another therapist and six weeks later after discharge from the practice with a fully rehabilitated fractured thumb, he called to ask me out.

That was eleven years ago. In that time we supported Lee through surgeries, chemotherapy, radiotherapy, wigs, return to work, good days, bad days, her return to Perth, my wedding, her wedding and two gorgeous pink babies for each of us which she was able to do having by then been seven years cancer free. Finally a survivor.

It was a year after the Field of Women that I learned over the email about Leanne's second cancer. Different boob, different type of cancer. Prognostically much better than the first, she assured me, and easier this time having done it all before. She was still tough.

I rang her and wept. She had softened though. She wept too.

In March last year, she was in Melbourne for a course on positive beliefs and life threatening illness. We had lunch. Things were wobbly with Simon. Having had her second confrontation with mortality, Lee wanted a seachange – sell her busy private practice, move to the beach and focus on her family. Simon was apparently not so sure; he was settled at work and at home and didn't want more disruption. Maybe that was because he had had his second dance with her cancer too. His priorities focused him in a different way.

We wept again. Her new boobs were booked in for April Fool's Day. I questioned the wisdom of this. She laughed. We had both worked in the medical model for years so knew that for surgeons to operate to reconstruct was an optimistic sign. We also laughed about the saying, 'Something good comes of everything'. Because of her illness I had met my wonderful Patrick, was now married, and our beautiful babies had by then turned three and five-years-old. Leanne took full credit.

Later last year I had another email explaining that the mystery of her back pain problem was answered. The cancer, the easier diagnosis to beat, the lesser devil of her two cancers, was all through her spine. Things were grim. I wrote back.

**From:** Katie Flannigan
**Sent:** Tuesday, 15 September 2009 8:27 AM

**To:** 'LR'
**Subject:** RE: A Bombshell (sorry)
Dear Blonde Bombshell,
Didn't catch my emails yesterday and have just read yours and I am not very happy about it.
Just sniveled thru a call to Patrick and the keys are all blurry, excuse any typos.
Won't bother you with a snively phone call from me right now as I anticipate you may be under siege fielding hundreds from others.
You must all be exhausted from tears and talk. Will give you a call in a few days.
I can't even imagine the conversations you are having with Simon and the Girls, it must be horrendous.
When I think of all that stuff I just cry and cry it's not fair on you, on Simon and on those two angels.
So so so so so so sad.
You know you have my love and support and am at the end of the phone and email but I am such a Virgo I can't help but think practically too. If you are heading east for hellos and goodbyes you are welcome to stay at Club Flannigan, the house, pool and garden are finished and we have a spare room for guests and heaps of room for trundles and rollouts, two busy young 'distractacons' for your two equally busy girls with lots of toys and fairy pink stuff and as of the weekend two baby bunnies for cuddling. You guys could come and go as you please. Resident babysitter provided :-)
You could take over the whole of the basement and be pretty self-contained. There are grown up quiet areas if you need space or be part of our home if you need company.
Depends what you need but you know what I mean.

Sometimes a hotel is great to escape too, I understand.
Offer is there; please consider it and I promise not to cry every time you come up for a coffee.
I am off to cuddle my girls as soon as the school bell goes and my big guy when he gets home, as I am sure are you. Bugger it.
Lots of love, thinking of you and I am serious about having you to stay for as little or as long as you like.
If a gathering of your friends and their kids would help, we are happy to host. We can turn the spa and BBQ on and you are away, chef provided (I use Paddy all the time :-)).
Lots and lots and lots of love,
Katie

**From:** 'LR '
**Sent:** Wednesday, 16 September 2009 10:18 AM
**To:** 'Katie Flannigan'
**Subject:** RE: A Bombshell (sorry)
Katie thank you so much. You are always so generous and of all people your emails make me cry (that's a good thing) because you are so supportive and caring. We may take you up on your offer just have to look at the timing ...
Will keep in touch.
Love Lee xx

I subsequently called and left messages that she never returned. I cried and cried. At night in bed the tears would come, silently and relentlessly. They came from a well so deep I could not articulate the emotion or the thoughts. It distressed me incredibly thinking about what it must be like for her. It was confronting. *There but for the grace of God go I.* A human tragedy so close and so real it was raw.

As any mother would, I knew she would be trying to set things in order for her little angels who would grow up without their mum. What if that was me? Would I write letters that they could read later when they were older? Make videos telling them how sorry I was not to be there and how much I loved them and that I would watch over them from Heaven, trying to present a positive image for them to remember? Write one hundred birthday cards each for the rest of their lives? Buy their eighteenth, twenty-first, and wedding presents, wrapping them in paper that would fade by the time they opened them? I could not imagine what she would say to them. What do you say to a three and five-year-old about concepts that their little minds can't even process? Anticipating lonely dawnings over their lifetime of special moments where a mum is needed for love and support or wisdom and understanding. Being unable to ease their pain or share their life's joy. Knowing that as with a last breath there would have to be a last cuddle, a final kiss goodbye. Their mummy whose job it was to protect them was going away and not coming back. What would she say to Simon? Awful awful awful.

Then this email from Simon.

**From:** 'Simon'
**Sent:** Friday, 20 November 2009 11:37 AM
**To:** 'Undisclosed Recipients'
**Subject:** Leanne
Sadly Leanne passed away last night at around 8pm. She was peaceful and in my arms with her family around her.
Thank you all for your ongoing support and sympathy.
Please at this stage no phone calls until Monday and please

no flowers.
Thanks again
Simon

Leanne had just turned thirty-eight. She was bald in her birthday photos.

Last weekend I took my two beautiful girls to stand on the turf of the MCG in the 2010 Field of Women. I tied knots in their bright pink ponchos because at four and six-years-old the ponchos were far too long. One size did not fit all. They made people smile that had heavy hearts and sad faces.

I was there on behalf of four people: Lyn the founder of BCNA; Gillian, one of my dearest friends and recently diagnosed; Geraldine, from my Mothers Group, also recently diagnosed; and Leanne.

I was once told that friends belong to us in one of three ways: they either come into our lives for a reason, a season or a lifetime. Why is it that those who have the most impact on our lives can be those we have lost? Being inevitable, mortality illustrates to us at an intellectual level how precious relationships are but when death is close to home you feel the visceral imperative not to take them for granted. In this case a 'reason', the trigger in a cascade of events leading to a life partner and family for me, a 'season' of life lessons ended or just a 'lifetime' of friendship too short.

# To Be Alert

*Beryl White*

Following extensive surgery for a breast abscess some fifteen years earlier, I'd gotten into the habit of self-examination. I had residual scar tissue in the breast, which presented as distinctive thickening over a large area, and. I was encouraged to self-examine because of the abscess. After fifteen years this had become routine. It was while on a conference interstate I discovered the new lump. I was alarmed, but had to wait two days until I got back to Melbourne to see my GP.

He tried to be reassuring and booked me in for a biopsy the next day. Following the biopsy, I was meant to return for the results two days later, but got a call from the surgery to come back at once. The GP was so concerned by the biopsy result, which indicated I had an aggressive form of cancer, that he had arranged for me to visit a surgeon that afternoon. The surgeon booked me in for an operation the next morning. From the initial visit to the GP, to surgery, only three days had elapsed. In a way I was glad they didn't give me the chance to stall.

The surgeon outlined my options, including an eventual reconstruction, and advised me that radical surgery was my best choice. He collaborated with a plastic surgeon so their aim was for a positive outcome medically and cosmetically.

Events had overtaken me; I was faced with a million thoughts, a degree of selfishness and grief at what had happened. The family was still coming to terms with the catastrophic result of a motor car accident in which my husband suffered major head injuries. I was now the only breadwinner, and I had an overwhelming need to be made whole again. In hindsight this proved to be a motivating factor for me to draw on every positive reason to overcome this.

\*\*\*

There was no time to waste. The operation was, as I was expecting, extensive and involved removal of all of the lymph glands under my arm.

At first the area resembled a piece of badly sewn corned beef. I was not prepared for the level of pain in my elbow, and that there was none in the wound itself. There was temporary loss of function in my right hand, with not enough strength to even hold a teaspoon. Much later after discharge I had a series of exercises to do walking my hand up the wall and each day trying to reach higher. I made this into a contest with one of the kids. Even then, doing my own hair with my right hand took many weeks.

My surgeon sat by my bed soon after I woke up to tell me that he was so confident about having removed all the cancer and the glands to which it had spread that he could not justify subjecting me to further treatment. He did not recommend either chemotherapy or radiotherapy.

Postoperatively the most surprising thing was the development of lymphedema, which causes retention of fluid and gross swelling. At first this happened across my back. Later, though, I had a minor injury to one finger, whereupon my whole hand became twice its size. Once this subsided all was well but it has been a minor inconvenience over the years. It can reappear even now if I exert myself by lifting heavy objects.

The mastectomy wound healed quickly, but the scar tissue was very sensitive, particularly to cold. Because I was expecting to have reconstructive surgery relatively soon, I created my own prosthesis. It was made by cutting small pieces of very fine fabric from an old t-shirt, and then was enclosed in a small pouch which filled a bra cup. This was both soft to wear and easily laundered. Later I made one to fit my swimsuit, so that normal summer activity resumed too. Apart from being asymmetrical, at times, I felt I walked a bit sideways. But these were small considerations.

***

Details of the reconstruction were discussed postop with the plastic surgeon. Usually this is done many months later. But because my own tissue was to be used, this surgery could be brought forward. The outcome, as promised, was that I would be back to work on full duties within eight weeks. My own tissue meant there was no chance of rejection.

The surgeon outlined the procedure, which looked much like a feat of engineering; the remaining breast was to be subdivided and extended, to be inserted in the area of the opposite armpit. A pedicle was to be fashioned and the rest of the tissue was to be attached to the site where the breast had been. Nerve endings and blood vessels were to be transplanted and allowed to develop over a five week period. An extensive range of sutures held this all together, which presented a challenge as to how I might live modestly with one enormous boob. An enterprising friend created a one cup masterpiece which was remarkably efficient and comfortable. This allowed me to sit out the next weeks easily.

All activity was restricted as I was not to extend my arm away from my body. My children who were at a high school nearby were able to come home during recess to assist me with meals. We had a very small kettle which I could just manage to make myself a cup of tea in the meantime. Housekeeping and housework was at a minimum or ignored for the duration.

As promised I returned to hospital for separation of the pedicle which had successfully achieved the transplanting of relevant blood vessels and nerves. From this, the surgeon created two breasts, so a semblance of normality was restored. I recommenced work on full duties, on time as promised, and I was allowed to drive again. Psychologically this was enormously positive.

In each instance when I was about to undergo surgery I was so impressed by the information given to me about what might happen and what to expect when I woke up. Whether it was from the doctors, the charge nurse, or even the hospital porter, I was told about drainage tubes, IV lines, and extensive bandaging. I told one doctor how good it was that there were no nasty surprises, and he said the object was assume I was uninformed about each step of what I would go through. This was why all staff had this responsibility to educate me.

I was monitored for the next five years on a very

regular basis, including mammograms, which I must confess I did not like much.

In a deep recess of my mind there was always the thought that one day my good fortune would end. To date, it is thirty-one years of thoughts.

Probably the most significant message I want to impart, is that self-examination is as important as other tests. Prompt action is vital, faith in those who do know what they are doing is necessary. It is okay to be devastated as long as that is put in perspective too

I received a great deal of support from my friends, the teachers at my children's schools, and valuable input from the nursing staff. I consider one should never underestimate the value of a casserole dropped off to feed the family. In case you wonder where my family was, well, I had no sister and my parents were recently deceased. But the world is full of wonderful people.

# My Mother, Myself

*Jacinta Thomson*

It was 26 June 1997. I remember the date well. It's a date I couldn't forget if I tried. I was in the waiting room of Royal Melbourne Hospital and I just wanted this appointment to be over because I had to get back to work.

I glanced up at the walls and was a tad miffed that they had advertisements for breast cancer – even though I was at the breast cancer clinic. It had not occurred to me that this was where patients would be diagnosed or leave their appointment with good news and never look back. I was certain that I was going to be one of the latter ones.

'Thomson, Jacinta,' my name was called out and I stepped into the room that was pointed out to me. My doctor walked in a few minutes later, followed by a nurse. After a quick 'hello, how are you?' the doctor began reading the file notes and the nurse – Fiona – introduced herself and we engaged in a bit of small talk. She was young, probably in her late twenties, but there was something about her that gave her an air of experience. Instinctively, I knew I liked her.

The chatter came to an end and there was silence in the room. It would have only been a few moments but it seemed a hell of a lot longer. I looked to Fiona for the next cue and her expression gave me an uneasy feeling, which was confusing because it still had not occurred to me that this situation could turn out to be devastating. I had a lump, nothing more, and nothing less – a lump that had been there for a year and should probably be taken out. I looked at the doctor who was still reading and he must have noticed the silence because he turned abruptly to face me. His expression was identical to Fiona's.

The moment of truth came. I had a diagnosis. My thoughts scrambled. My words were a mixture of statements and questions almost falling over each other.

'But I'm only thirty. That doesn't make sense. People don't get cancer at thirty, do they? How can you tell that it's cancer?'

Tears were falling thick and fast and my sentences were barely audible. Then it occurred to me in an instance that did not resemble clarity – not even sprinkled with a tiny bit of clarity. Words fell over each other as the adrenalin kicked in again.

'Oh,' I said, feeling very sure of myself. 'You have me confused with my mother. She's the one with cancer. They told us she has two weeks to live but that was three weeks ago. She was bleeding internally and they don't know where it's coming from and ...'

I stopped and I turned to Fiona who had her mouth and eyes wide open. She closed her mouth to talk but it was the doctor who spoke next.

'Jacinta, we have the results of *your* biopsy here, but let's talk about your mum. What hospital is she at?'

'John Fawkner Private,' I said.

'And what type of cancer does she have?'

'Liver,' I replied.

Fiona moved towards me and took my hand. I had begun to realise that I was the one who was confused and was trying to get my head around the facts. My mother and I had been diagnosed with cancer in the same month but we were being treated by different doctors in different hospitals.

More tears followed and more disbelief and again I tried the *but I'm only 30* line followed by, 'Do you think I can take a day off work? I might go to the pub and have a drink.' It was the first time I saw my doctor smile that day.

I stopped off at a pub for a drink. I had to work out if I should tell my parents that I had cancer or if I could go through it without anybody knowing. After all, Dad had just found out that his wife of many years had cancer and was going to die. Surely he didn't need to worry about me too. I decided to visit Mum and Dad and get some sort of safe feeling.

The house was empty, which was strange because Mum was always in bed and Dad had taken some time off work to get hospital stuff sorted for Mum. I called up work and my boyfriend to give them the news. As I put the phone down, it rang and I answered. It was Dad and he had gone to work. He told me that Mum was in hospital getting a blood transfusion. I asked Dad why he was calling his own house when he knew that nobody was there. He said that he didn't know why but he had a feeling that he had to call. Up until then I still had not decided on whether or not to tell them my news but in that split moment I couldn't stop myself. The words were out before I knew it. Silence followed. I had to say something quickly to reassure Dad that I was going to be okay. I had no idea if I was or not but I knew that Mum needed Dad more than I did.

'I'll go and visit Mum in hospital then,' I said.

There was no reply.

'Dad, did you hear me? Is it okay to visit Mum at the hospital?'

There was another delay but he finally spoke. This time his voice was shaky and he tried to compose himself. 'That's a good idea. I will meet you there'.

Mum greeted me with a huge smile and tears running down her face. She would have hugged me had she not been hooked up to monitors and hospital gadgets. Dad was already there. He looked very pale and moved like he had been punched in the stomach. He made his way towards me to give me a hug. He had just received an almighty shock, the second one for the month. His wife and daughter were fighting cancer.

The months that followed were hard and tiring. Mum's doctor had finally located the position of her blood loss. Her situation was no longer the two week sentence we had gotten originally. The doctors did not speculate a timeframe for her or for me so we plodded along doing the cancer thing together. We had our treatments and I hated every single minute of mine but I knew, I just knew, that I still had to be there for Mum and Dad.

Mum sadly passed away in 2002. It is now 2011 and even though my cancer experience was not an easy one, I have a different outlook on life. It probably sounds like a tired cliché but it is true – for me, anyway. I love the simple things. I love listening to my daughter laugh, I love feeling the rain on my hands, I love feeling the temperature changing when you move into the shade and I love listening to the church bell chiming. Ask me if I regret the year of 1997. A few years ago I would have said yes but today with confidence I can say absolutely not.

# Rollercoaster Ride

*Kim de Koning*

To be told you have cancer
to have numerous operations and
radiation treatment
five days a week
Is like being on a rollercoaster
With all the ups and down

pain / family / heat / support /
peeling / love / tiredness /
kisses / fear / friends / sadness
and poetry
like a kind hand on your shoulder

Made the rollercoaster
a lot easier to ride

# Told the Words

*Kim de Koning*

when told you have cancer
Your mind says to itself
I have cancer
I have cancer
I have cancer

body as cold as a grave stone
you feel a cold breath
on the back of your neck
And wonder

# Where There's Life

*Sarah Black*

Late in the afternoon, the phone rings.

'Hi, honey. I've just finished with Barney. Guess what? They've shrunk by half! He said to crack open some champagne.'

My mind rears in turmoil. I knew Mum was seeing the doctor, but I didn't allow myself to think much about it. We were, to be frank, both secretly expecting bad news rather than good. She's been having some odd, maybe worrying side-effects recently. But this! This is totally off-the-scale fantastically good news.

'Oh Mum, that's wonderful! Shall I put a bottle in the fridge? Come and have dinner with us.'

Soon they are here, my brightly clad mother and her protective helpmeet, my father. The little boys tumble over them, puppy-like. They are too young to comprehend the details, but understand tumours as 'little balls inside Granny's body that aren't meant to be there'. They know we are happy because the little balls have gotten smaller. I hug my mother, and rejoice in the flesh on her bones.

Way back at the beginning we feared cancer, but perhaps even more so, we feared cancer treatment. Memories of my grandma's cancer journey, twelve years previously, were fresh enough. We remembered the pain she suffered, the searing nausea, the weeks spent on the living room couch vomiting into a bowl, the loss of a loved one inch by inch, as the chemotherapy poisoned her and the cancer slowly ate her up. She said, philosophically, in the beginning, 'Oh well, if the worst comes to the worst, I've had seventy-three good years.' And in the end it did come to the worst. The fragile little bundle of bones finally gave up Grandma's ghost, and she was gone. It took about three years. So yes, we were afraid. More of the suffering than of the end – years of affliction followed by a death that was too soon, and yet not soon enough.

Mum's journey with breast cancer has, then, been longer and more full of life than we could have imagined. From the discovery of a lump through to today, it has been a decade. First of all, after diagnosis, came a year-long grab bag of treatments – chemotherapy, surgery and radiotherapy. These were interspersed with counselling, beetroot juice, and lifestyle courses on how to wind a turban around your bald head and recreate the memory of your eyebrows with a pencil. She lost twelve kilos and took on the translucent pallor of the ill. She smelled (I never told her this) like an experimental laboratory, like a pharmacy, like a sackful of chemicals. Which she was.

There was pain, though less than we might have feared. Dad and I, again, were the watching ones, trying helplessly to help, but this time Mum's role had changed from supporting cast to lead actor. She was the one who had to pass through the valley of the shadow of death. There can be no companion on that journey. But Mum wanted to live, and she lived in hope. I was shocked by her bravery. Luckily she is strong – not sporty but tough, made for endurance.

After the year of aggressive therapies came follow-up Tamoxifen and all the rest. Then, for several years … nothing. Nothing at all. Test after test for breast cancer markers came back negative. You beaut! Each passing month felt more and more like a new beginning. Our fears slowly receded. We dared to believe it was gone. I went to live overseas and Mum, who loves travel above everything, came to visit and buzzed around Europe like a dragonfly in a sunny garden. I had my babies and came home again. Mum's blood tests continued to be clear, and we breathed deep sighs of relief as we got on with life.

Unseen and unsuspected, though, the cancer was doing just the same. Slowly, slowly, it recouped, after all the treatments and excisions and other onslaughts were over and done with. Quietly it burgeoned, its presence screened by the continuing litany of 'clear' blood results. Its urge to live was strong, just like Mum's. Cell by infinitesimal cell, it grew and prospered, pushing aside the working parts of Mum's body to make room for itself.

One otherwise uneventful day, about two years ago, Mum became ill. The doctors said it was flu. I wasn't worried about cancer. Mentally and emotionally, we had long since left its shadow behind. I should have been worried about it though, because that's what the illness turned out to be. Not swine flu, but metastatic breast cancer in the lungs and liver. Many tumours. Big ones, some of them. All those blood results of the intervening years didn't actually mean much at all. They were data gathered in good faith and according to the dictates of current science, I know. But from a non-statistical standpoint, from the standpoint of a husband, a daughter, a friend, they were irrelevant, misleading rubbish written up in reassuring medicalese. The limits of knowledge.

Suddenly, just like that, the silent assassin had declared its hand again. The size, number and location of the tumours meant that neither surgery nor radiotherapy was feasible. When we heard the extent of it, we were ashen with horror. The pit that had been in my stomach eight years before suddenly opened up again, a deep and horrible chasm. Mum felt like a dead woman walking. I just hoped she would survive the few months to Christmas. We have seen others be taken that quickly. We all, quietly, thought that the last chapter of Mum's story was beginning.

And yet, and yet … medicine seemed to have failed Mum, but the little black bag has some pretty remarkable tricks in it these days. We thought we knew the cancer game, but there were treatment options we had never dreamed of. In the short time we had been away, having our Indian summer of good health and busy years, chemotherapy had changed profoundly again. Doctors and drugs had become even cleverer at cheating cancer of life and limb. Now, Mum's life seems to be the prize in a game that is played between drug companies and the Grim Reaper. Amazingly, the drug companies are winning at the moment. And not only are they keeping her alive, they are keeping her well.

No more days of pain and boredom in the hospital. No more putting up with the headscarves, wigs, and sidelong glances of strangers in the street . Now Mum takes her chemo at home, in tablet form, and goes on living. She gets tired and delicate, but she bounces back.

She still has her hair – and her eyebrows and lashes. And by God, the tumours are shrinking.

It hasn't been seamless, of course. She is fragile, and some side-effects are uncomfortable and unsettling. There has been a lot of trial and error, a lot of oncological knob twiddling, to get regimes and dosages right. Even then, there is a certain element of serendipity involved. Nobody knows exactly what will work, or how well, or how long for. The rules of the game keep shifting further and further onto the side of the drugs and doctors, but cancer is still a disease which thumbs its nose at the human desire for control.

Cancer wants to take my mother but, thanks to the whim of these drugs, I've still got her. At least for the moment. We have learned – *are* learning – to focus our joy on today. Tomorrow can come another day. People talk about cancer as a 'fight', and perhaps it is. But it seems to me more like a gamble, a roll of the dice. For our family it has been a journey, one we have been on unwillingly but one which has taught us to appreciate the privilege of one another's company, and to refrain from courting unhappiness. It has also shown us what a deep wellspring of hope is within us.

Glasses poured – a bottle of bubbly for us, lemonade for the little ones – and a toast! To Mum's robust constitution. And to the doctor. And to the miracle medicines he provides. And to the good fortune to get cancer in the twenty-first century, not before. Tumours shrunk by half! This evening we'll wallow in our happiness. The little boys can't believe their luck, having fizzy drink before bedtime. Mum can't believe her luck, that she's here to see them. And that there's still more life to be lived.

# On Finding Myself Alive

*Jenny Sinclair*

Five years.

Say it.

Roll it around in your mouth and in your mind.

Five years. It's not forever. But it's not a short time. It's not nothing.

It's long enough for a child to grow from a helpless baby to a streetwise urchin, or from a sweet primary schooler to a surly teen. It's the kind of time handed down by judges for medium-sized crimes – large thefts, the infliction of non-fatal injuries.

It is, in other words, a considerable chunk of any life.

No project should take more than five years. It's long enough to require serious work, depth, intensity, endurance. If something took less time – a year or two – one might suspect one was getting by on nervous energy, clever tricks, a single good idea, a lucky break. More, and the whole thing might become a drudge, an endless highway. Five years is long enough.

My project, finished today, 1 July 2010, was surviving. Not-dying. I achieved it, as most long-term projects are achieved, one step at a time.

Five times 365 (plus one for a leap year and one for luck) daily hormone-blocking tablets.

Five times twelve equals sixty abdominal implants of another hormone-blocking drug, each involving a trip to the GP.

And before that, because this project really took five and a half years, six months of assorted chemo, surgery and radiotherapy treatments.

Just the usual.

While one is engaged on such an all-important project, there is rarely space for reflection. And to my grim determination to pile day upon day, to put one step after the other without tripping over the single word 'recurrence', add this: that I had to walk that tightrope without looking down. That I could not think of death, because I did not want to catch its eye. That I set myself the task, as the days and weeks went by, of living a good life; of being a good mother; of writing; of using the body that had betrayed me to wrest as much *life* out of life as I could – small things like a bike ride every morning, a swim in cold water every afternoon, and big new things, like learning to surf (badly) and learning to swing on a trapeze (even less well).

That I did these things without grace or skill was not at all the point. Once, when I was fifteen, I won a long-distance running race through sheer bloody-mindedness; the sports teacher had explained to us how to breathe our way through painful 'stitches' – take deep, slow, regular breaths, and keep on running – and I applied the advice, sailing past faster girls who were doubled over with the hurt in their abdomens. I may not be the quickest, the best, or the most stylish at what I do, but I am tenacious.

I get it done.

So, I travelled. I studied. I taught. I queued at the supermarket and I cooked and I let myself spend hours looking at art. I went out to shows, and I worked in the garden. And it was all good. It was all life. But I never took my eye off the calendar; a year, two and a half years (the halfway mark), three years, four years (only one to go), six months to go, one month, one week, one day.

Today.

My doctors tell me some women get nervous at this point. Some women feel that the drugs have been keeping them alive, and worry once that safety net is whisked away. A month ago, I chose to have a CT scan and bone scan. It was a tense and tedious morning of medical activity to one end: to give reality to an affirmation I'd made more in hope than in belief in late 2004 – that my body was now clean, clear and strong.

That the disease was gone.

What I face now, at the end of five years, is something other than fear. It's the return of a future; not the positive-thinking, it'll-be-ok, Pollyanna plans made when the odds were fifty/fifty, but a real future, as reliable as a future *can* be. On this cold Victorian day, crouching over the coffee table in front of the fire in an old house not far from Castlemaine, scribbling in my notebook, I can finally say: I won't die. Not yet.

And there's the thing. Five years pass, and I'm forty-five. I was diagnosed at thirty-eight and a half. I was youngish, a new mother. Death was not of interest to me.

Now I know what menopause is like. I know what it is to be disfigured. I know what it is to be disabled. I have permanent injuries – small, easily concealed, but I must take care. I have a more-than-theoretical sense of what five years is. My concept of time has been altered. I counted the days forward, rather than simply looking back and saying, 'That was five years ago.' The idea of my days being numbered makes perfect sense; now, you could give me a number of days, and I could picture exactly how long that was.

So I know what it is to believe in death. My long-lived family go before me. I can expect, now, many more healthy years. I can hope, even, for another child (as the medicine that saved my life has saved that hope too). But I will die, one day.

And there is so much to do. Today, stepping from the counted days to the uncounted, I feel beset by choices – books I want to read and write, friends I want to drink with, gardens I want to plant, cities in India I long to see. There is so much in this wide world, and even between the walls of this old house, first and foremost being a child of six, who is asleep in the next room. Ten lifetimes? Give me twenty.

Lately, I've been having moments of clarity; not only a sense of anything being possible, but also of my right to choose what that thing will be. My illness has translated into a new kindness to others, and at the same time, a new impatience. I know now that everyone has some struggle, visible or not, and I try to remember this when I'm out in the world. But I also suffer time-wasting and the pressures of society to be and do certain things less gladly. This, I know, is because my life is now mine in a way it wasn't five and a half years ago. I have *earned* my life: it was bloody hard work to keep it, and no one can tell me what to do with it.

This may fade. Maybe I'll go back to wasting time, pottering, doing less than I could, going with the flow. And maybe that's only human. But now, with the fire roaring red and the clouds hanging low over the soft green hills, I feel at the centre of an ever-expanding whirl of possibilities. And to begin, I will put down my pen, step outside, and like a newborn baby, feel the shock of fresh air rushing in.

# Omens and a Tunnel

*Robbie Wesley*

The day before the operation, my car died. It turned out that I had let the water in the battery cells run dry, and that I needed a new battery. Still, the symbolism was a bit disturbing.

On the morning of the operation, I tried to turn my computer on to send a last minute email. The computer made a horrible noise, flashed unusual lights at me and refused to function.

Another bad omen.

The night before, I had rung my pragmatic and completely insensitive German friend to let him know I was about to go into hospital. 'Uh huh,' he mused. 'Somebody, I don't remember who, said their mother died under an anaesthetic, before they even started to operate.' I wondered why he thought it necessary for me to have this information.

They wanted me to check in at eight am, so another friend drove me to the hospital. She accompanied me to reception. 'I'm making sure you don't run away,' she said.

If I'd known what was ahead of me, I might have.

It had been almost two months since I had tried on a low cut, sleeveless top and checked it from different angles in a change room mirror. My heart plummeted;

there was a definite indentation on the edge of my right breast. It had been a 'dimple', which had alerted me to the presence of cancer in my other breast two years earlier. I had been listening to a program on the symptoms of breast cancer on Radio National while getting dressed when I saw it. It was directly above the nipple, and easily detected by an ultrasound. The doctors had persuaded me to have it cut out, and strongly recommended follow-up radiation therapy.

I had my doubts about subjecting my delicate tissue to further trauma before I had checked with my favourite oracle, the *I Ching*. The translation of this ancient Chinese manuscript, also known as *The Book of Changes*, is consulted by throwing three coins six times and noting the pattern of heads and tails while keeping a question in mind. I seldom do anything important without taking account of its august wisdom. This time a moving line (Hexagram 44, first line) told me:

> *It must be checked with a brake of bronze ...*
> *If one lets it take its course, one experiences misfortune.*
> *Even a lean pig has it in him to rage around.*

The explanation went on to say, 'If an inferior element has wormed its way in, it must be energetically checked at once ... If it is allowed to take its course, misfortune is bound to result; the insignificance of that which creeps in should not be a temptation to underrate it.' Upon this unequivocal advice, I rushed to sign up.

I didn't want to go through all that again. This indentation was very peripheral. Maybe it was just a fat crease? I'd had my yearly mammogram only six months before, and had been declared clean then. But I made an appointment with my doctor, just in case.

The first time I was diagnosed with breast cancer, I had allowed my mind to descend into a state of almost constant fury at the behaviour of a housemate who obviously had serious problems of his own. I was living in a situation I had been promising myself to get out of for several years. When I told the news to one of my friends in Northern New South Wales, the New Age capital of Australia, she said, 'Cancer! That's a wakeup call!' I tried to take this on board, and, indeed, changed my external circumstances radically for the better.

But the mind has habitual pathways and is harder to reprogram. Overcoming repetitive negative thought is like trying to walk through the worst kind of clay mud in ripple-soled boots. Even when you manage to extract a foot from its clutches, with a horrible, sucking, squelching pop, the clay, with its embedded pebbles and matted grass, clings in a heavy wad to your boot, while the other foot has sunk deeper.

I was going through another period of furiously angry mind when I discovered the second indentation. To begin with, I was in a situation which is not uncommon among the daughters of farmers. Having handed the farm over, holus bolus, to my one brother at least a decade earlier, my father was now working his merry way through the inheritance our mother had always promised her daughters, but which, now she was departed, we discovered she had neglected to mention in any will.

I was seething because a Government department had conned me into buying a car and leasing a flat as a home office after I had successfully answered a totally mendacious advertisement for a part-time worker; twenty-five to thirty hours a week, which is all I felt prepared to undertake. Instead, the first week, after a fortnight of gruelling training, took sixty hours, though I was only paid for twenty-six. This included six hours of unpaid time trying to get their computer, their answering machine and even their telephone into some kind of working order. Lies, damned lies and statistics. I could feel my blood pressure rising.

I was disappointed because, following this debacle, I had been retrenched from two assistant teaching jobs in high schools, which I had been led to believe would last longer than a single ten-week-term each. In fact, this was probably a blessing, as the kids were so out of control in both places that I felt unable to be much use anyway. Altogether, my mind was not in a happy place.

A secondary cancer is far more life threatening than a primary. When the margins and sentinel nodes were declared clear on my first cancer, I became almost cocky.

'I've been lucky,' I declared to anyone who would listen.

A bald-headed, yellow tinged, emaciated lady in the radiation waiting room said to me sourly, 'It can come back, you know.' Almost as though she hoped it would, just to show me. If it comes back, it usually means that the cancer has spread, and you don't know where it will go next, or how long you've got left.

I became convinced that I'd had my chance and blown it. I was to be punished for my lack of control over my mental processes. This time I could possibly die. In the many weeks it takes to get a diagnosis in Darwin, I tried to turn my mind around, in the hope that if I managed to do so, all may yet be well.

My GP felt that the dimple was too lateral to worry about. Barely on the breast at all. Still, just for peace of mind, she wrote a referral to the diagnostic imaging people for a mammogram and ultrasound. It would be two weeks before they could fit me in and another two before the results would become available.

I carried on with normal life while I waited, but I did not have the confidence my doctor seemed to have. There had been those recent *I Ching* readings with moving lines about knives, blood and dragons fighting. All I had been asking was if I should move out of my flat. At the start of the year, a Tarot reader had let me choose a card from his pack. He had predicted, ominously, that this year 'something would have to be cut out.' To cap the bad omens, my stove started oozing blood and smelling of singed flesh on the very day that I bought new saucepans. Probably the karma of a skink had intersected with mine, and it had committed unwitting suicide by being in the wrong place when I turned the stove on, shorting the system, but it was like something out of *The Exorcist*. The electrician never came, and I couldn't cook for days.

On the drive to the hospital, we heard on the radio that Jane McGrath, the high profile cricketer's wife, who worked tirelessly for breast cancer support, being, herself, a victim of the disease, had just died that morning.

Because this was my second episode of breast cancer, the doctor had ordered a bone scan several days before the operation. It was to take place in a part of the public hospital where I needed to turn up immediately after admission on the big day. Radioactive dye would be injected into the breast to locate two sentinel nodes. I was very determined to have this procedure because if, upon removal and testing, these nodes are shown to be clear, it means the cancer has probably not spread, and no further lymphatic clearance is needed. Losing more lymph nodes than absolutely necessary can cause a whole raft of problems which I strongly wished to avoid.

The nurse who admitted me was new. She insisted that all my preoperative procedures were to take place in the private hospital which is connected to the public hospital by a tunnel. Along this tunnel I obediently, though somewhat dubiously, went. I sat in the waiting room for an hour before being called in to the room where I had my original mammogram. The staff there knew nothing about radioactive dye. They warned me that if I went back to the public hospital to find out, I would be returned to the end of their queue. Nevertheless, panic drove me back along the tunnel, as I didn't know how long the dye needed to travel before they cut me open.

The radiologist in the public hospital had, indeed, been wondering what had become of me. Yes. I had been supposed to check in with him upon admission. Here was the dye, ready for me in a massive syringe. We had to make our way immediately to mammography so that he could see exactly where to inject it. Back through the tunnel we raced.

My breast was squished into a pancake shape for the next three quarters of an hour, during which I was given a fifteen centimeter long injection of local anaesthetic, a wire was inserted to guide the surgeons in their forthcoming excavation, and the all important dye was finally administered. A bit shattered after all this, I staggered back along the tunnel and sat in the sun to recover. After I'd thawed out for a while, I thought I'd better check how my time was going. I asked a passerby, who discovered, to his obvious surprise, that his watch had stopped. Another omen.

Back inside the hospital, I found my way to the wrong reception area. The sister in charge rang around to find out where I was meant to be. After the third call, she put the phone down in a hurry. 'Quick. They're looking for you all over. You're meant to be back in the other hospital to have your dye checked.'

'Are you sure?' I asked. They had said nothing about having to come back.

The sister was sure, so once again, back along the tunnel. Stood in a queue. Notified reception of my presence. They didn't want me. More phone calls. No. I was supposed to be in radiography in the public hospital. I was getting very familiar with that tunnel.

Yes. The radiologist had to locate my nodes with the dye *before* my operation. This was different from my first experience, when the surgeons had traced the path of some blue dye while I was anaesthetised.

Afterwards, I was put to bed for the next few hours. I think they were scared of losing me again. In the next cubicle, a red-faced young man was being encouraged to fart, loudly and explosively, by a gaggle of giggling nurses.

'Come on,' they said. 'This is probably the only time in your life you'll ever have a woman happy to hear you farting.'

I spent my time reading a Buddhist book on the impermanence of the body. I reviewed the life I suspected I might be leaving and, in spite of its difficulties, I felt floods of gratitude for all the wonderful experiences

I'd had. I remembered how, on my walk the previous evening, a feather had wafted out of an empty sky and hovered in front of me. Obviously an angel was keeping watch. I thought, *Even if I die this time, it doesn't mean the angels have stopped loving me.*

\*\*\*

It was very dark and peaceful as I started to emerge from the anaesthetic. I was aware of someone periodically taking my blood pressure. Around the third time, I asked how it was.

'It's a bit low,' she told me. 'One hundred over sixty.'

The next time it was ninety over fifty. Then eighty over forty.

*I could just drift off,* I thought. *Just let it sink to nothing and be out of here.* Weirdly, it felt like an opportunity. It was, after all, what I'd been building myself up to accept. The thought of escaping was seductively attractive. After all those omens, I didn't doubt I had the choice. But then a kind of curiosity got the better of me. The story lover's perennial *what happens next?* and I thought, *Plenty of time for that. Might as well stick around for the next installment.* As though I'd come to a good place to finish the book, but if I wished, I could go on and read the sequel.

I chose the sequel.

I asked for a cup of tea, read a stressful article in a *Time* magazine, and managed to raise my blood pressure to something resembling 'normal'. With all its inevitable future complications, I decided to embrace the rest of my life.

# Cancer

*Robbie Wesley*

This pretty little planet.
Diamond waters sparkle by forested or sandy shores.
winged creatures grace the air.
Seasons. Stormy grandeur. Sunset glory.

I may be leaving you soon.

Fickle, sickle, pale moon blooms and withers
as I have bloomed. And wither.

Once innocent, I fashioned daisy chains
and crowned my childish self with future hope,
and lay, spread eagled, on grass cushioned slopes
and knew myself
                    upon
                                my Mother's breast.

This poisonous little planet.
Orphaned children wail their murdered parents,
land-mined limbs;
their sisters raped, then beaten for their shame.
Wanted kids, unwanted kids, proliferate.
This little orb is bursting at the seams.

She groans, and heaves, and tries to rid herself
with floods and feverish droughts.

My Mother's breast is cancerous.
As is mine.

I may not be sorry to be leaving you.

# An Extraordinary Life

*Melissa Petrovski*

One of my earliest memories is riding my older sister's twenty-four inch pushbike down the road outside of our home. My feet could hardly stretch to the pedals. It was a new experience to me as I rode down our street with the wind in my hair. It was a great feeling. Suddenly, I catapulted straight over the handlebars as the front wheel jerked. There I was flat on the bitumen, knees grazed, and winded; that was the end of my bike riding escapades for a while. I have experienced many moments in life which have resulted in a downward turn one way or another, either physically or emotionally. I have the scars to prove it.

Life has not always been kind to me and I have struggled to succeed and maintain a balanced life. I was raised in a family of seven children and having left school at an early age I worked for most of my life. I moved out of the family home at seventeen-years of age and into my own flat. I matured very early in life. I have been through relationship difficulties and at times raised my children on my own. I have lost two brothers in-law to cancer. More recently, four years ago, my mother passed away and two of my adult children suffered serious health issues.

I was blessed one year after my mother's death with the birth of my grandson. There were mixed emotions at this time – grieving the anniversary of the death of my mother combined with the anticipation of the birth was certainly a challenge, but my grandson is a precious gift to me.

I was where I wanted to be in my career. I knew who I was and I had established a positive self-image. I had recently become a registered psychologist and I felt that professionally I had achieved a great deal. I was proud of the counselling practice I had established and the type of work I was engaged in. I have an interest in assisting people who have an intellectual disability and have always worked in a career helping people for over thirty years. I had worked hard and achieved a combination of five degrees and diplomas, including a Masters in Counselling. It took me many years to attain the qualifications I earned. I felt like I had finally reached the peak of my career and my life.

Then cancer invaded my body.

I was diagnosed with advanced breast cancer on 18 March 2010 at fifty-two years of age. It started in the middle of the night months before. I felt a small lump in my right breast. The next day I went to my doctor of many years who gave me a referral for an ultrasound and mammogram, which I underwent that week. It was the usual practice of the surgery I attended to phone patients if the doctor needed to discuss test results and another appointment would be scheduled. There was no call from the surgery.

When I attended a subsequent appointment with the doctor for another medical issue, I enquired about the test results and the doctor said, 'We didn't call you, did we?'

I replied, 'No, I didn't receive a phone call.'

The doctor stated, 'Then everything must be fine.'

I asked the doctor to look at the results and he briefly glanced at the file on the computer screen. He then told me the lump was only a blocked duct.

I enquired, 'Well, what do you do about a blocked duct?'

He replied, 'You don't do anything about it'

That was it. Nothing to be concerned about according to the interpretation of results, so I moved forward with my life relieved I did not have cancer.

***

I had experienced mastitis and fluid in my breast when breastfeeding years before and the sensation in my right breast was very similar, so it made sense the symptoms could have been a blocked duct and it would clear itself eventually. I had also experienced over the years lumpy breasts and all the previous mammograms and ultrasounds came back clear so this was not unusual for me.

The surgery had destroyed the mammogram and ultrasound films as they have a policy of destroying them after one month if uncollected by patients. This made it difficult for any follow-up at a later time. At no time did the doctor examine my breasts.

As time went on I questioned if there was something wrong but the doctor's determination that there was no reason for concern reassured me that everything was fine. This failure to further investigate, concluding there was nothing serious wrong, continued to feed my own self-doubt and I suppressed any negative thoughts or concerns about ongoing symptoms, reassuring myself the doctor had to be right.

As time progressed I had a few other pressing medical issues to attend, but when the issue about the breast did not go away I returned to the doctor and again told him I was still experiencing problems and I would like to see a specialist. My return to the doctor was the result of a conversation I had with a friend who told me that a breast specialist could aspire the fluid out of the breast with a syringe. I was pleased with this discovery. By this time the symptoms had increased to what I could describe as a thickening inside the right breast and then, in time, pain in the breast. The doctor then referred me to the breast specialist and I expected that the fluid could be syringed. I could not have been more mistaken. The breast specialist examined both breasts and my armpits, and said, 'I am so sorry to have met you under such terrible circumstances. This is very bad, very bad indeed.'

I thought this could not be happening to me. I did not immediately comprehend what the breast specialist was saying. She did not say I had breast cancer but I could sense the urgency in her voice and her body language was that of extreme concern. Surely the breast specialist was mistaken and it was some kind of error.

The breast specialist advised me to stay at the breast unit and undergo several tests later that very day. She had arranged an appointment for a mammogram, ultrasound and biopsy. Alone and desperate I went into a state of shock and confusion. I could not remember the time I needed to return for these tests.

After several visits to the toilet because my body was in shock I finally managed to leave. I phoned my family for support and waited in my car close to the breast unit for my husband to meet me. I rang my boss and informed her briefly of the situation and asked her to cancel my appointments at work for the following Monday.

My husband arrived and my family collected my car. I waited to undergo the procedures as instructed. By the time the mammogram, ultrasound and biopsy were completed I knew something was terribly wrong. These tests were thorough and extensive.

The specialist who performed the biopsy enquired, 'Has the surgeon spoken to you about chemotherapy or surgery?' The radiographer had also mentioned to me when she was scanning my armpit and chest that she was checking to ensure the cancer had not gone through my chest wall or to my lymph nodes.

A nurse then said to me, 'I know it's hard but try not to worry over the weekend.'

There was a lot of silence during the procedures, although all of the professional team appeared so concerned and were very comforting. I left at six-thirty at night. Everything in my life changed on that day. It had been my day off, I was happy and all I wanted was advice about fluid on my breast.

I returned home to face my son and two daughters and explain to them as best as I could what had been explained to me. I felt terrible to have to share this news, as if I was shattering their happiness. I was sure I had cancer and even though they attempted to reassure me, they sensed something was terribly wrong and they too were extremely concerned.

Given a choice I would never undergo serious medical tests on a Friday. It is such a terrifying waiting game to wait a whole weekend for results.

Following this distressing weekend of anxiety the next appointment on the Monday confirmed the breast specialist's prediction: breast cancer – a 7.5 cm tumour. I showed the breast surgeon the results of the previous mammogram and ultrasound. She remarked that those results certainly did not indicate a blocked duct. The breast surgeon said that she could tell I had breast cancer when she examined me and recommended surgery to remove the right breast. Further tests were immediately ordered to ensure my body was able to endure surgery and to determine if the cancer had spread.

I didn't understand most of what was going on. I rang my boss and asked her to cancel my commitments for the rest of the week at work. The next day I returned to undergo further scans of my body and undergo blood tests. I had never experienced scans such as these.

During the CT scan I was injected with a dye as I lay in a machine that was round. My arms were strapped and I needed to stay still. I went in and out and was instructed by a robot voice to hold my breath. I was told I would experience strange sensations and I may even feel like I was losing control of my bladder. The bone scan takes quite a while to complete as well.

I attended the next appointment on the Thursday of that same week with my brother as my husband was sure the news would be straightforward and he was required at work. The prognosis provided devastating results. The breast specialist stated, 'I am sorry. I cannot save your life. The cancer has gone too far.'

*Time limited* was the term the breast specialist used – a term which has come to replace *terminal illness.* She told me I had advanced breast cancer as the cancer had spread to my bones. She then explained the type of breast cancer I have is oestrogen positive, which means the cancer feeds off the oestrogen. I pleaded and bargained with the breast specialist to save my life. I was so desperate I told her I didn't care if I lost the breast. I just wanted to live.

Although the breast surgeon understood my urgency all she could do was explain how she could remove the breast and lymph nodes. I asked the breast surgeon how long other people had lived with this type of breast cancer and whether there was any hope.

She replied, 'Some of my patients have lived five to ten years with advanced breast cancer.'

I then commented, 'So I need a bucket list.'

She agreed I did, concluding I was not going to live a long life.

I was then instructed to undergo further bone x-rays to ensure my bones were not about to fracture. This time it was a straightforward x-ray to my limbs and hips.

The breast surgeon was very efficient and arranged for an oncologist that very afternoon to attend to my medical needs and to provide me with the medication to suppress the oestrogen, strengthen my bones and thereby prevent the cancer from spreading to my organs.

The oncologist reassured me that treatment was available and that I was not living with a death sentence, even though the breast surgeon had said the cancer had gone too far. The oncologist accessed the results of the bone x-rays and reassured me my bones were not about to fracture.

Surgery was scheduled. I chose to go to the public hospital as my medical insurance had lapsed. I waited one month for the surgery as I was already on medication to suppress the hormones. Also, because the cancer was already advanced, I was informed waiting for the surgery wouldn't make a great difference at this stage.

That day my most beautiful and precious granddaughter was born. After another long day I put all the devastation aside and went to the hospital to see her. I also phoned my boss and concluded I would not be at work for that month or for weeks following the surgery.

Many questions entered my mind. Why me? How could this happen when I had my life mapped out? There was no history of cancer in my immediate family, I took care of my body, I had regular mammograms and ultrasounds, I conducted intermittent breast self-examination; I had attended my general practitioner on a regular basis and requested investigation of presenting symptoms, and I understood the basic information regarding breast lumps.

I did not, however, have extensive knowledge about breast cancer. All of the medical terms presented to me were so unfamiliar: oestrogen receptors, metastatic breast cancer in the bones, medium aggression. It was all too much to comprehend and process. I was inconsolable and cried every day. I could not sleep or eat. If someone close to me phoned, I cried; if someone called in, I cried. I just wanted my life back.

I came to understand in a short period of time that breast cancer was a sinister invasion that immediately and intensely disables any sense of control over one's own life. Cancer torments one's sanity in a manner which is unimaginable on a daily basis. My mind was still reeling from the diagnosis. I needed to find the strength to go through with the surgery and the treatment.

The day of the operation arrived exactly one month following diagnosis. I said goodbye to my family and prayed as I was wheeled into a small room next to the operating theatre. The anaesthetist gave me a pre-med which allowed me to sleep, a reprieve from the thoughts that rushed through my mind causing me to panic. If I was unconscious I did not have to consider what was about to happen to my body. It would never be the same again.

I was asleep for a while and then woken by the surgeon who instructed me to sit up. She drew with a marker on my body mapping out the surgery. I lay down again and was wheeled into the operating theatre where a mask was placed on my face and I was soon unconscious.

After the operation, I was wheeled back to my room where my family were waiting. I later found out they all cried when I went into theatre.

I soon realised I took everybody who loved me with me through the experience: my husband, my grown children, my siblings and nieces and nephews, and all my friends. Knowing it affected all the people who loved me was not an easy burden for me to carry. Not only was I hurting from cancer and the operation, but also the suffering of my family.

After four days in hospital I was discharged. The post-surgery recovery was extensive. I needed so much help and support to be able to cope firstly with the ordeal of the surgery, and then with the recovery.

I was fortunate because my family rallied around to help. When I was discharged a family friend came to my home every day to shower me. This friend agreed to shower me because my family had difficulty comprehending what had happened to my body and were unable to look at the disfigurement. Home nurses came every day to measure the fluid draining from my body and to change the drainage bags. I was in contact with a breast nurse prior to and following the operation; she was available for advice when I needed it.

The breast surgeon also continued my care by attending to me at the outpatient appointments. I hated the outpatient visits as I did not like to see the patients who were wearing head wraps due to hair loss from chemotherapy. They were a reminder they had a better chance of survival than I did. I enquired why I was not having chemotherapy; the breast nurse told me it was because the cancer had already spread and the specialists were not trying to cure me.

During one of the outpatient appointments there was a discussion between the surgeon and the oncologist as to whether radiation would be beneficial. The breast surgeon wanted me to have the radiation as further tumours could grow and further complicate my prognosis even though the oncologist believed the radiation was not necessary.

I decided to take the advice of the breast surgeon.

I was fortunate enough to go to a private radiation service and it was all fresh, new and modern. For five weeks I attended five days per week. The radiation oncologist was thorough as he explained the process of the treatment. He took the time to show me scans on his computer of the cancer in my bones and explained to me the extent of the cancer in my body and where the tumours were located. This was the first time I saw the scans. He said he was going to read out the results and I asked him to refrain from doing so because I had already read the report and it was distressing. He was so kind. He only revealed the information I needed to hear because I had heard the poor prognosis too many times and it affected my ability to stay positive.

During the radiation treatment I was terrified by the whole process, including the machinery and the effects of the treatment. I was alone again, as I had been during the previous medical tests and surgery. The machinery was large and white. I was placed on a tray with what looked like a large globe that would rotate around my body. During the first appointment, I was again scanned and my body was tattooed to mark where the nurses would align my body to the machine. These tiny tattoos had to be re-inked on occasion as they faded. Regular scans were also taken of my body to ensure the nurses were accurate in their measurements. A heavy gel sheet was placed over my chest every other day; it was cold and clammy.

The radiation oncologist was wonderful and supportive and all the nurses were very caring. One day the nurses played Celine Dion through the speakers and tears rolled down my face. I am pretty resilient but I did mention to the nurses they may like to carefully choose the music for that room, as it was a great alternative to the ongoing daily silence.

Toward the end of the radiation treatment my chest on the right hand side burned and blistered. All I could do was to stay at home and nurse my wounds, except for the times I needed to attend the radiation sessions. The breast nurse at radiation oncology advised me on treating the burns. I cut down singlets into tubes to cover my chest as little as possible; I wore a sarong around my waist and treated my wounds with a burn gel until the burns healed, which took approximately three weeks. Nothing could touch those burns, they were so painful.

Following the radiation and when the burns had healed and the scarring had settled, I was fitted with a breast prosthesis. I felt this was the best option for me rather than breast reconstructive surgery as the breast surgeon explained that recovery would be more difficult if I were to undergo reconstruction at the same time as removing the breast. I needed to focus on my recovery so reconstruction was not my priority. Choosing not to undergo reconstructive surgery means the scar and the removal of the breast is a daily reminder I am living with cancer.

An appointment was arranged and I went to see someone trained in fitting the prosthesis – the government funds one per removed breast every two years. This prosthesis also meant I needed to be fitted with bras that were designed to hold the prosthesis so new bras needed to be purchased.

With the surgery and radiation complete and prosthesis fitted, I was ready to take an active defence against the cancer. I chose to fight for my life with every resource and strength I had at my availability. Cancer is not something you can run away from. Treatment is an ongoing process.

I have a monthly injection called Zoladex and daily Femara tablets, both designed to suppress the oestrogen, and daily Bondronat tablets to heal my bones. Every three months I undergo a blood test and every six months I undergo the CT and bone scans to determine if the cancer is managed.

Sometimes, it feels like a waiting game to determine not if but *when* the cancer will attack the organs. It is gruelling to undergo these tests and have to wait for the results. The issue is whether there are cancer cells circulating in my system and, if so, it may be a matter of time until the cancer cells cluster to form cancer elsewhere. Rather than be negative, I try to view the need for the tests as life-saving. The oncologist told me I will never be told I am cured but he did say, 'It appears you are here for the long haul.' So far the results have been positive, indicating the bones are healing with no further progression of the disease.

I also realised after I was diagnosed I was not satisfied that conventional medication was enough to fight this disease. I wanted to give myself the best chance at recovery. I commenced researching treatment options that included complimentary therapies that can assist with a healthy lifestyle.

As I was taking an active role in my treatment, I went to see a psychologist to help me challenge my own self-destructive thoughts. I went to see a naturopath and an integrative medical specialist for advice regarding daily nutrition. I visited a reiki healer who helped me with spiritual growth and inner peace. I have learned to meditate and relax. My diet maximises my chances of good health. I have a multitude of daily vitamins and complementary therapies which include daily juicing and a healthy eating regime. Healing my mind, body and spirit became my number one priority.

Rather than succumbing to the doomsday prediction of my future – or lack of – I found out that not all women die early of this disease, but instead survive longer than expected.

***

My life has not always been an easy one but that is what life is all about with all its discoveries, challenges and ups and downs. My experiences helped me grow, develop and emerge, become complete and strong. People have the ability to be whoever they want to be if prepared to accept the challenge and to work hard.

The cancer has not robbed me of who I am and if I can achieve so much in my lifetime, perhaps I can also overcome this disease and remove its powerful force. I can say I am at peace with myself. I would encourage others not to allow life's challenges to stand in the way of success and enjoyment, and do not allow anyone or anything to crush your spirit.

We have two choices in life: to endure or give up.

I always take the first option – choose to be strong, positive and death-defying. My belief is that people are dying every day for all sorts of reasons so death and dying is no surprise. It's part of life. All people die; it is simply a matter of timing.

I am learning it is so essential to live to the fullest, have fun and maintain a good sense of humour. None of us know what can happen in the next moment or the next day and so it is so important to enjoy each moment and to be close to the people we love. Our body is a very fragile gift of which we must take the utmost care.

I read once that our body is our temple; I think this is true and life appears so short from where I am standing.

We are only provided one chance to make the most of this lifetime and so I will be embracing this opportunity with the strength and vitality that keeps me from surrendering and the courage to keep fighting.

I love life; I intend to continue with this journey. There will be no death sentence for me – not yet anyway. When death does invite me I will accept the challenge gracefully and with the utmost dignity I deserve.

I do not need to hold my prognosis before me like a ticking bomb. Most days I try to take time out from the constant reminder I am living with cancer just to be me and enjoy my day. I have days where I just don't do cancer. It is so important not to live life as a cancer patient, but as a person who lives with cancer.

# Introducing Bertie

*Neridah McMullin*

Meredith stood facing the sea, inhaling deeply. She swivelled her feet from side to side into the squeaky sand, sinking deeper and deeper until her ankles were completely covered.

The waves gently peeled off and long smooth folds crumpled along the shore.

A south-westerly was blowing down on the beach, and out amongst the elements was one of the few places Meredith felt truly calm. She was a solitary figure on the beach this morning but her reverie was soon broken by the manic barking of her dog, Bertie.

Bertie was a six-year-old Jack Russell. Meredith didn't believe she had ever known another dog quite so disobedient. He never did what he was told and was completely incapable of following commands. But he was so endearing to her. He was wonderful company and he followed her everywhere. And he would smile at her. That's what won her over every time.

She could see him up ahead, skipping along in shallow water, yapping loudly. He was a muscular, stocky little dog with short stumpy legs. A favourite past-time of his was chasing seagulls. Relentless in his pursuit, he never looked close to getting them. He probably wouldn't know what to do if he did.

Meredith hoped he wasn't chasing the Oyster Catchers – her favourites. They were striking looking birds with black bodies and white markings on their chests, bright red beaks and matching red feet. They were graceful in action and bearing. Upon take off, they'd run in fast, neat little steps before they took flight. And then there was their soulful call that haunted Meredith. It always made her stomach drop to her feet.

Oyster Catchers were also territorial birds, and came back to the same part of the beach every year with their chosen mate for life. Perhaps that's why Meredith loved them so much. She had also chosen a mate for life. Or more accurately, she and Will had chosen each other. They were sixteen when they'd met, and they had been inseparable for forty-four years.

Will had had cancer and after the tumour had been removed and chemo endured, he was given the all clear. But within days he'd developed an infection: an insidious bacteria that couldn't be halted, and he died suddenly overnight of 'complications', septic in her arms.

She had been furious with the hospital, the oncologist and all the other specialists. It should never have happened. Will won his fight; he was still meant to be here, with her, so they could live their lives together.

Upon Will's death, she raged. She withdrew entirely from their world. There was a panicky-welling up in her chest and she often found herself overwhelmed. She preferred to do different things in this different life she'd found herself floundering in. She shopped at different shops, ate at cafes her friends didn't know and drove to places via a different route. It just made it easier to get by.

Meredith's daughter called every day, just to say 'Hi.' She kept calling and Meredith told Celia she just needed time. They had a close relationship but there was always a reserve between them.

Meredith was horrified one day when Celia made the comment to her over coffee of how jealous she had been of her mother's relationship with her father.

'Celia, darling, what on Earth can you mean?' Meredith asked. 'Your father loved you, I love you. Your father adored you.'

'Not as much as he adored you, Mum.'

Meredith strenuously denied it. Then after a few weeks thinking about it she realised for the first time what it might have been like for other people outside of them. It had been an all consuming love and they knew it. Cocooned and precious, they were devoted to each other.

Had they excluded their daughter?

'I knew you loved me, Mum. I just sometimes felt left out because you and Dad were so close. You didn't seem to need me like I needed you. You were the most smitten couple.' Celia smiled. 'It was sickening. I couldn't get a look in either way.'

'Celia, I don't know what to say. I'm so sorry, darling, I had no idea we excluded you. It was not a deliberate act. I thought you were a happy soul.'

'No, Mum. I wanted more – from both of you.'

'I'm so sorry, darling.'

Meredith was still crying when she got home and she kept on crying at the most ridiculous things. She stepped in one of Bertie's dog poos and walked it through the house, unknowingly trampling it into the carpet in the front hallway and all the way into the kitchen.

Retching as she cleaned it up, she put the news on to hear about the latest load of illegal boat people arriving in Australia who had to be held in over crowded detention centres. This news was followed by three stabbings in the city, followed by the floods in drought-stricken Queensland that were washing everything away.

Meredith howled some more and decided to go to bed. She thought she could still smell Will on the sheets and she'd reach out and feel where he'd once lain, imagining him there again. It was silliness but it always helped her fall asleep.

In the morning, Meredith spoke to Celia, who admitted to feeling better after talking it through and having a cry. Meredith felt better, too, if a little puffy-eyed and so she headed out for her morning walk.

Bertie's frantic chasing and barking was the background music to her thoughts. She looked up and saw another lone person walking along the beach towards her.

*Oh God, it's Clare Aubrey.*

Clare and her husband Charles had recently moved to Port Fairland. They were young retirees – like the rest of them – but Clare was unwell with breast cancer and the move here was obviously meant to be a recuperative one.

Clare was good looking. No, she was better than that. She was beautiful. She looked like she'd wrinkle her nose for sure but she wasn't a snob. She was a real surprise. Clare changed the mood of a room; the atmosphere shifted around her.

At drinks after golf last week, though, Meredith decided she didn't really want to be too friendly with them. They had way too much in common.

As soon as she'd met Charles she knew he wanted to talk to her about Clare's illness. She could tell by the way he sought her out, his intense eye contact and his forced nervous, sympathetic smile.

*Go away,* she had wanted to say.

'I think you and I have something in common,' Charles said, leaning in close.

'Well, it's certainly isn't our golf handicap,' Meredith said in an unfriendly tone. She was an excellent golfer.

'No, that's true. I meant cancer.'

*Jesus Christ, I don't want to talk to you about this.*

But talk he did and soon Charles had Meredith cornered next to the bar for half an hour. She was sure Clare would have been mortified if she knew how much Charles had told her about her cancer and prognosis.

'I'm terrified, Meredith,' he whispered. 'What can I do? What am I going to do?' His voice cracked.

'Get a grip, for God's sake, Charles,' she said to him. 'We're all terrified.'

Meredith gulped her glass of wine and ducked and weaved out his way to get free. She walked home light-headed, not wanting to think about Will or Clare or anyone else's illness. She just couldn't go over old ground again. She needed time. It was all still so raw and tender, and way too present for her in her new life.

Meredith avoided golf this week but at bridge she heard that Clare and Charles had been invited to join on a new table.

*God strike me down.* She knew it wasn't very generous of her. Her attitude went against every grain of her being but she just needed privacy. She was still in mourning.

Bertie was now a long way up ahead. Meredith could see him jumping up and down in front of Clare and running around her in frantic crazy circles.

Meredith pulled the collar up on her coat, as the wind was bitingly cold.

'Is this your dog?' Clare asked as Meredith got closer. She saw the recognition in Clare's eyes but Meredith refused to look back at her, pretending to call her dog instead.

'Yes,' Meredith answered, wanting to keep on walking.

'What breed is he?' Clare asked.

'He's a Jack Russell.'

'He's an energetic little guy,' Clare said, moving in closer. 'I'm Clare. We've met briefly a couple of times. Meredith, isn't it?'

'Yes, that's right. Come on, Bertie,' Meredith called.

The wind was blustery and as the tide was sneaking in around them they had to run up the beach to stop themselves from getting wet.

Meredith turned and was facing Clare just as another gust of strong wind buffeted them.

In slow motion Meredith watched in horror as Clare's blonde wig rose slowly above her head. It lifted and hovered above her momentarily before swooping and swirling and blowing away with the wind.

'Oh no!' Clare wailed. Pale bony hands grabbed at her bald head where the wig used to be.

Meredith was rooted to the spot, fixated by the patchy blonde straggles of fuzzy hair that had somehow defied chemo. Will's head had looked like that too.

The wayward wig tumbled and twisted in the wind before it floated gently down, landing into the sea not fifteen metres from where they were standing.

'I'll get it!' Meredith yelled as she moved with an agility she'd thought long gone.

But she was too late.

Bertie was a quick as lightning. His little legs paddled hard and his head was the only thing left submerged. The wig was getting wet and quickly started to bob below the surface as a wave tumbled over it.

With a mouth full of sea water, Bertie grabbed the wig and somehow, coughing and spluttering with the wig still in his mouth, turned and headed back towards the shore.

Meredith called to him.

'Good boy, Bertie. Good dog, bring it to Mummy.' Meredith thumped both hands on her legs to encourage him to come to her.

But Bertie had other ideas.

As soon as Bertie's legs touched the sandy bottom of the shore he shot off at right angles down the beach. He hit the sand running and bolted like a jet propelled engine. Every now and then he turned his head to smile at them with the wig still firmly in his mouth.

'BERTIE! You little prick of a dog! Get back here now. Do you hear me? Come here this instant!' Meredith screamed. 'Oh God, Clare, I'm so sorry, I'll buy you another one. I am so, so sorry,' Meredith panted.

By this time, Clare was crying.

'BERTIE! BERTIE!' Meredith screeched.

Tears were now streaming down Clare's cheeks and

her eyes were squeezed tightly shut. She was bent over and looked ill.

Gasping for breath, Clare said, 'Your bloody dog. Has just taken. My bloody. Six hundred dollar wig!'

'Oh, Clare. I'm so sorry,' Meredith said, as she saw out of the corner of her eye, Bertie trying to shake the life out of the wig.

Then Meredith recognised something.

The rhythmic shaking of Clare's shoulders and the way she was gasping for air.

She wasn't crying.

She was laughing …

Clare's tears were tears of laughter. Hysterical, guffawing, hearty laughter.

With relief, Meredith started laughing too and they both ended up in fits.

'It's from Russia, you know,' Clare said. 'It's real hair.'

'Oh, that's disgusting,' Meredith said.

'It is, isn't it? I hate the bloody thing.' Clare said, lying on the sand quietly. 'Charles likes me to wear it.'

'I understand,' Meredith said.

'I'm dying, you know.'

'I'm sorry,' Meredith whispered.

'Your husband died of cancer, didn't he?'

'No. He died of complications from an infection he got in hospital. Before he got it, he was in remission,' Meredith said.

'Really?'

'Yep. He beat it,' Meredith answered.

'I really need a friend right now. Someone I don't have

to pretend in front of. Someone I can talk to and swear and say it like it is.'

The two women smiled at each other.

Standing up, they were just brushing the sand off their jeans when Bertie appeared. In his mouth was one very bedraggled, sandy and saliva-encrusted wig. He dropped it at their feet and sat proudly in front of them, puffing and smiling.

Meredith and Clare looked at each and burst out laughing again.

'I've got a beanie in my pocket if you'd like to wear it,' Meredith offered.

'Yes please, it's freezing!'

And side by side, the two new friends continued their morning sojourn up the beach, flanked by a little dog yapping and barking ahead of them.

***

*This is based on a true story.*

*Names and places have been changed to protect and respect privacy.*

*Clare won her battle with breast cancer and still enjoys golf and bridge and long walks on the beach.*

# The Pillow

*Sandra Simpson*

The sunlight shone through the bedroom window of my first floor flat where I lay on the floor soaking up the warmth. I began to doze off. As I was drifting in and out of sleep, in a relaxed state of awareness, sounds would arise and fall away, such as a distant siren, a bird singing, a ladder being manoeuvred on to the window. I vaguely thought that someone had come to clean the windows until there was a loud rapping on the glass. I raised my head and saw a paramedic looking at me.

'Are you all right?' she said with urgency.

'Yes,' I replied sleepily. 'I must have dozed off reading my book.'

'Could you please come down?' she requested. 'Just to check that you are all right.'

'Sure,' I answered. The sleepiness had cleared somewhat. I got up and I walked slowly down the flight of stairs.

There was a paramedic and another woman standing waiting.

'Your neighbour could see you through her window and thought that you had had a heart attack,' she said in a calmer tone of voice.

I looked at the woman standing nearby with shoulder

length wavy brown hair. She had a very concerned look on her face. I had never seen her before.

'You weren't breathing,' she said as I wondered what she was doing looking through my window.

'I was breathing,' I said. 'I had just fallen asleep while reading a book.'

'All right then. We are glad you are all right.' They departed.

This sort of thing had been happening quite often. I had been dozing in the park and people had come up to me to see if I was all right. I contemplated my response and decided to be grateful and polite as it was good that people looked out for the wellbeing of others.

\*\*\*

Native grass swayed in the breeze and a willy wagtail fanned its tail nearby. I sometimes wandered up to the remnant red gum grassy woodland in the park to do some gardening.

'You look thin,' said a woman whose house looked onto the park. She was a nurse and we regularly had a chat.

'Actually I have a lump in my breast,' I replied. 'I had better get it seen to.' I had had previous lumps in my breast that had turned out not to be a problem. The lumps had been smooth and sore but this one felt like a chocolate crackle. It wasn't sore.

It hadn't gone away.

\*\*\*

I was fed up waiting for the doctor's rounds. I was still a smoker and had run out of tobacco. I hauled myself off the bed and told the nurse at the front desk that I was going home to get some more tobacco and before she could say anything I was gone.

'Where are you going?' asked a nurse who was looking at me with a smile on her face. I noticed that there were only two of us in the lift.

'I'm escaping,' I replied.

'You had better press the button for the ground floor then,' she said and departed as the doors closed shut behind her.

I lived close by and was a little puffed and sweaty when I returned and lay back on my bed. My angst had disappeared and I didn't even feel like a cigarette. Soon a nurse entered my room – the one that I didn't get along with very well.

'Where did you disappear to?' she said, staring at me.

'Home. You have kept me in here longer than you said and I ran out of tobacco so I went to get some supplies.'

'You are not meant to do things like that. Give me your pillow. I am confiscating it. It's the hospital's property now. This is your punishment.'

I could not believe it. I felt upset and wanted a cigarette now. How dare they take my pillow! It seemed that I had missed the doctor's rounds for when I returned from smoko the doctor had arrived.

'Sorry,' he said apologetically. 'There was an emergency.' A smile lit up his handsome face.

This, of course, made me feel teary and I explained what had happened and how the nurse had taken my pillow and had no intentions of returning it.

'I'll get it back for you,' he said with a smile.

He felt like a hero to me. I think I was falling in love. I

think I had a fever. I don't think that it was a type of love fever; I think I had an infection. The doctor removed the drainage tubes and said that I could go home. I packed my bag and went straight to the pub and ordered a double shot of whisky to ease the pain. I couldn't roll a cigarette and I began to sniffle and then cry. The barman refused to give me another whisky, so I went home.

Once at home I placed the pillow under my arm where my breast should have been but now there was just a big wound full of stitches and lots of pain and there was also a tissue expander. This was to stretch the skin for a later breast reconstruction. It was made of plastic. This may have been a problem as I was a greenie. Maybe my body was rejecting it. My thoughts returned to the nurse who had taken my pillow.

With beads of sweat on my forehead I went downstairs and kicked the small curved pillow all the way back to the hospital, into reception and it just lay there, still. Alone, I returned home feeling pleased with myself.

I had to attend the breast clinic on a regular basis. The waiting room would be full of glum faces. We would wait and wait and then the doctors/surgeons would make a grand entrance looking like they had just stepped out from the pages of a Mills and Boon novel, clean cut, well pressed suits and with an air of sophistication. They wanted me to take a certain medication. However, I had found out that a possible side effect was uterine cancer. I refused to take it. Things seemed to change after this. I felt that my views were not being taken seriously. I sure had fallen out of love.

I was on the public hospital waiting list and was awaiting elective surgery to have a permanent breast implant and reconstruction. But I had begun to have my doubts about the benefits of cosmetic surgery.

My views were also changing. I believed there was a disproportionate amount of emphasis in Australian culture on body image and sex. I was also around fifty-years of age and had many interests and hobbies. I had been having saline injections into the tissue expander to stretch the skin and I had begun to feel a little like an inflatable doll on a torture rack. Then I discovered that there would be future operations, one for a nipple and further operations for replacement of the breast implant. There was a risk that the silicone may leak, that the implant could obscure the detection of another breast lump, and there were general risks involved in surgery and anaesthesia. I couldn't weight-bear with that arm and it made doing yoga quite difficult.

One day I received a letter from the hospital administration saying that I had been offered a place for surgery at a private hospital. It would not be the same surgeons though. I snapped up the opportunity. I attended a preliminary session with one doctor who was very kind and honest with me, explaining the risks very carefully and concisely. After seeing him I felt that I could no longer have the operation for the reconstruction and I rang the nurse and explained my feelings. She was very supportive. I had to see the specialist who suggested that I could have some fat removed from my stomach to create a new breast. He explained that it was quite a serious operation that would involve a lengthy stay in hospital and there was a risk of infection. I happily told him that I had decided to have the expander removed and he seemed a bit put out that he had made the visit to the hospital. It was just a small operation and I was back at home the next morning feeling happy.

I wondered what I would say to the nurses and surgeons at the public hospital and when I rang the nurse she had no idea that I had had the operation. When I went in to see the surgeons next they seemed annoyed.

'Why, didn't you like it?' the plastics surgeon said, looking slightly offended.

'My priority is my health,' I answered.

Finally, I felt empowered.

# Anointing

*Marlene Marburg*

Anoint
pink ridged skin
stretched across a rib cage
where breast gave life
and nearly took it.

We do what we can;
little, but enough to
damn undress a heart.

We peg our smallness
on unknown lines,
watch them flail and fold in.

We anoint with oil
the wounded places,
soothe with fragrance
silent as love.

Touch by tender touch,
we gently elevate
like pick-up-sticks,
unbending vows.

# An Unexpected Journey

*Mairi Neil*

This room is too small. A tiny desk jammed in the left corner as we enter through the door. A four-shelf bookcase laden with pamphlets melts into the right wall and four grey cloth office chairs cluster beside the desk, silent when moved against the carpet, which is another nondescript grey. I think how crowded the room will be when filled to capacity – patient with partner or friend, the doctor and a nurse/counsellor. Or, maybe cosy – it depends on what news is delivered.

Now, there is only Deb, the nurse who has been looking after me. We are waiting for the doctor to return and already I feel claustrophobic. The Venetian blinds are semi-closed on the pencil thin window but I can feel the chill from the stormy sky threatening hail.

I don't gasp for air, or take deep reassuring gulps. Instead, holding my breath, I almost stop breathing. Perhaps a subconscious plea for time to stop, even be rewound, will be answered. This morning has become surreal. I can sense rather than see Deb behind me, her chair close enough to be reassuring, or grab me if I lose control. I think she expected me to sit in the chair parallel to the desk, face the doctor and her, but I sit once removed, where a husband or partner should be. Where John should be. I suppress a mixture of emotions: anger, pain, sadness, self-pity, and fear.

The empty chair reminds me I'm widowed eight years. A silent voice in my head acknowledges reality – I'm fifty-seven, alone, and no man is going to find me attractive now. I tremble for a moment, an almost imperceptible jerk. Deb leans closer; I can feel the heat from her body and grit my teeth, willing the tears to stay behind burning eyeballs. The ache for John's strength beside me is making me emotional. I must stop thinking the impossible.

Dr Sarah returns, hunched as if warding off an arctic wind. She clutches several files to her chest. It has been less than a week and already I'm a paperwork headache for the system. She sees my raised eyebrows, smiles weakly and spreads the manila folders, obliterating the smooth green surface of the desk.

'Your GP will get copies of all reports and so will your surgeon.' She sniffs and apologises, 'I'm not feeling well – must be coming down with a cold.'

I murmur sympathies. So does Deb. Later I'll laugh at the irony. Three of us commiserating over her cold after she has told me I have breast cancer – Invasive Ductal Carcinoma Grade 2 breast cancer, early stages.

'… should only be a lumpectomy … probably some lymph glands. No results yet if it is hormone receptive, won't really know if it has spread anywhere else until the operation and more biopsy results … definitely radiation treatment, maybe chemotherapy to follow. Any questions?'

I don't know what to say so babble thanks, grateful for her expertise, her kindness, a health system that I hope will make me well, or at least do its best to make the route to oblivion as easy as possible.

I can see in her grey eyes that she is already preparing herself for the next patient. Three hundred women a day diagnosed with breast cancer in Australia – an epidemic Dr Sarah copes with by keeping women like me at a distance.

She leaves the room as quietly as she came in, a mouse-like figure, all fawns and browns, pale-skinned, fair hair lacking lustre because of her sniffles. I recall her cold, cold hands – petite, slender, surgeon's hands. She operates at The Alfred when she is not delivering bad news at BreastScreen Victoria.

I won't forget her part in my journey, her soft voice and her cold, cold hands. She'll remember me as Patient 061.52.72.

Nurse Deb is different. Although we have only shared a few hours, they have been intense and earth-shattering hours for me. We bonded over our love of elephants when she admired the pendant around my neck, a gift from John. I heard her sigh of relief when I did not break into hysterical sobbing or react angrily to Dr Sarah's news. Those stages of grief will come but my Scots Presbyterian childhood kicks in when I face trauma. I have learned to hide my grief, contain my anger.

'I'll visit the local swimming pool and give a primal scream underwater,' I say with a nervous laugh. Deb nods her approval.

'There's some more admin stuff.' Deb is apologetic and begins to usher me into another room. I struggle and stumble over the crammed chairs, I feel a stunned mullet expression has taken residence on my face. Training kicks in; Deb pauses. From her face, I can see her go through a checklist from her counselling course. She advises I stay in the room for a few moments, let the news sink in.

'It is a bit of a shock,' I murmur. 'I had almost convinced myself the biopsy would be okay – it would be a cyst, or fatty tissue.' Another silent practised smile and nod from Deb. I'm glad she has learnt sympathetic silence. I picture the days ahead when everyone will have a breast cancer story, unsolicited advice about what to eat, what to do, speculation about how I got it.

Emotion lumps in my throat. John was such a good listener; I ache for his comforting arms, the squeeze of his hand, the loving smile that twinkled in Paul Newman eyes only for me.

I shrug off my torpor. 'I'm fine, Deb. What's the next step?'

***

On the evening of Wednesday December 29, before the last chemotherapy session, daughters Anne and Mary Jane organise a celebration: the special food, Cinderella party hats and hooters reminiscent of childhood parties. The role reversal a reminder nurturing passes from generation to generation. I suppress a fleeting fear I may never see them be mothers.

The hat keeps slipping off my bald head – added entertainment to an evening introduced with their giggle-producing card, which featured a middle-aged woman complete with pearls, sitting in an armchair knitting what looks like a yellow scarf.

Her thought bubble: *Thursday already? Where does the time go?*

And text beneath: *Mary hurries to finish her boob tube in time for the weekend.*

Inside:

*To Mum,*

*The day has finally arrived!*
*It's your last* ~~birthday~~ *chemo!*
*We love you and are proud of how strong and brave you have*
*been through it all. You deserve a really big gold star!*

*Love Mary Jane and Anne xoxoxoxo*

A friend, Eva, arrives with belated Christmas presents, making a welcome addition to the party. She laughs at the hilarious good luck card, sharing our Pythonesque humour. We even joke about my steroid-induced swollen red face and hyped-up chattering. The girls agree, 'It's like Mum's on Speed.' They present me with an iPod Shuffle, a distraction for the hours hooked to the IV machine – a selection of favourite singers (Bob Dylan, Elvis, Neil Diamond, Judy Small, Carol King) already loaded. I'm blessed by how much the girls cherish me and amazed such a tiny machine holds five hundred songs. Anne had noticed my difficulty working out the different settings of the mp3 player my older sister had given me and decided an iPod Shuffle less complicated. I'll download meditations on the other machine. Cate's generosity will not go to waste.

Many people ring, email, or send text messages of good luck. They understand the importance of finishing chemotherapy in 2010. I really want 2011 to be free of major medical procedures, the New Year to be a renewal and return to normality – whatever the new normal may be …

When we arrive at Brighton, the Cabrini staff apologise. There's at least an hour delay in the Chemo Room – again – and the cafe onsite is closed. There will be a lengthy wait for blood test results too. Bloods go by courier to Cabrini Malvern Pathology, any advantage of less traffic on the road counteracted because of the rescheduling required by Christmas public holidays.

'That's okay.' I put the receptionist at ease with what I hope is an infectious smile. I am buoyant, want to share the joy. 'This is my last chemo and there is a whole street of shops two minutes walk away.'

Once involved in a cancer journey, you realise just how many others are travelling the same road. I know it will be a long day and insist my friends Barbara and Mary Jane don't feel obligated to stay too long – the iPod will earn its keep but they insist on staying until I'm hooked up.

We go in search of a cuppa to fill in time and choose a restaurant where Barbara's youngest daughter, Vanessa, waitressed when she was studying. Barbara observes, 'This decor has hardly changed in a decade but it's still popular.' She laughs.

Mary Jane is not surprised, 'Their ham and cheese croissants are to die for!'

Cancer patients and carers learn where to find the best food at best value – alternative places other than hospital facilities. The girls have checked out most of the nearby eateries, including the hotel – their refuge the night I had the emergency operation to remove the haematoma – and after the initial chemotherapy heralded my first 000 ride in an ambulance since my appendix burst when I was twelve-years-old! The memories of emergency surgery and pneumonia after my first chemo are still raw. I take a deep breath, luxuriate in the aroma of freshly roasted coffee and tasty raisin toast delivered by a cheerful waitress, her blonde ponytail a jaunty pendulum as she returns to the counter to collect Mary Jane's order. I savour the snack knowing within the week the chemotherapy will reduce my desire to eat and a metallic taste will leech the pleasure.

The blood results have not appeared when we return to Cabrini but the nurses find me an armchair – I've moved up the waiting list. The nurses are always caring, polite and pleasant despite their heavy workload. Staying overnight, and often the last to leave the Chemo Room, I observe the tiredness etched on pale faces. Each patient has individual chemotherapy instructions, some have Portacams like me, and others have PICC lines, or the IV inserted directly into a vein in the arm. Setting up individual sessions involves meticulous care of damaged or collapsed veins, discussing side-effects, double-checking the drugs and oncologist instructions.

The green gowns and gloves the nurses wear, the purple bin emblazoned with CYTOTOXIC WASTE are reminders it is radioactive poison. Mistakes have deadly consequences. I recall the warnings in the booklet issued at the start of treatment reminding me to flush the toilet twice as a precaution against exposing the family to whatever my system excreted.

Today, Phillipa and Jo share the load. A great team, they synchronise like a long-married couple while hooking me up, laying out paperwork, sterilised equipment, and prepared drugs on the trolley. Constant *beep-beep* echoes but they instinctively know what machines require attention without the need to scan the room. I never feel neglected or abandoned.

There is a treat because today is not my usual Monday. Valerie, a regular Thursday volunteer offers to massage my hands and feet. Silver-haired, retired and chatty, she peers over blue-rimmed glasses. We discuss books as her gentle hands, lubricated with body butter, knead and soothe. Barbara and Mary Jane prepare to leave. Mary Jane's plucked eyebrows form question marks. She shakes her head in amazement, and blurts to Valerie, 'You must have a magic touch. Mum hates anyone touching her feet.' Valerie pauses, gloved hand hovering over the jar of cream.

'Please, continue,' I plead and smile at my youngest daughter. 'This is different and feels divine,' I say.

Mary Jane grins.

Barbara voices our thoughts, 'It must be those relaxation drugs!'

'Better than whisky,' I whisper as I kiss them goodbye.

Valerie continues to massage and chat about her book club. She recommends *The Book Thief* and *The Guernsey Literary and Potato Peel Pie Society* and several other books that disappear into the fog of memory. I feel my eyelids droop. Jo agrees the books are great reads as she changes my IV bag – the Phenergan and Valium-laced fluid finished. My relaxed body now blasted with the real deal but I'll sleep through most of the treatment and always tell the girls to go home. I appreciate their support but I cope with the hospital procedures. Why disrupt their lives anymore than my illness has already? Sometimes trying to be sociable is stressful when I don't need company.

Valerie moves on and my eyes roam the room where I have spent many hours since the start of this journey. I may forget (chemo brain a much talked about and real phenomenon) and want to imprint the details. The hospital's effort to create a pleasant ambience is a success considering what happens here. Most people enter with mixed feelings: fear, dread, a dash of hope. The framed photographs hanging above each chair are of coastal scenes. Not a moody sea but calm and blue; there are palm trees, beach houses; peaceful seascapes to induce serenity. I recognise Brighton and Sandringham, even Port Campbell. Victoria has so many picturesque attractions along the coastline.

In contrast, the armchairs are nondescript grey-fawn leather with adjustable foot and head rests. Comfortable and functional, they have a removable side-table where volunteer Lorraine deposits morning and afternoon tea, lunch, and cups of water at regular intervals. Patient comfort and needs always priority.

The room is large with three sections divided by a half wall and reception desk incorporating the nurses' station. There is a fridge housing bags of blood for those needing a transfusion boost. (When I had pneumonia, I was grateful for two bags of blood to boost the recovery of my white blood cells!) Fresh flower arrangements and a string of Christmas and Thank You cards decorate the counter today, plus two large hampers with a sign advertising a fundraising raffle drawn in the New Year. I buy tickets but don't expect my luck to change!

Silver-grey trolleys earmarked for each patient stand at attention in the centre of each section, their sides decorated with black garbage bags, a canary yellow sharp needle dispenser, and the purple bin for the plastic tubing and bags of toxic residue. Fellow patients recline in the chairs, a mixture of ages and sexes – and cancers. Breast cancer patients are identifiable by their painted nails; the drug company advising dark nail polish protects finger and toenails from damage. My first three sessions I wore gothic black but today the polish is dark red in honour of Christmas. During treatment, I don black cotton gloves and insert my hands into large frozen mittens until the mittens defrost, which takes about an hour. Not everyone submits to this painful procedure but the discomfort is a small price to pay if it saves my nails from dying or permanent damage.

I wear a bright red shirt to match my Santa-suit complexion caused by the heavy dose of steroids required before, during, and after the chemo. Along with the glowing face, I feel and look bloated. One of the reasons I fall into a deep sleep rather than just relax with the Phenergan is because the steroids cause insomnia (and in some cases an insatiable appetite). I never sleep the night before chemotherapy. An ironic laugh escapes when Jo tells me, 'If you take the tablets after lunch rather than after dinner they don't cause insomnia.'

If only I'd heard that advice before my first chemotherapy session, not my last! Several of the patients are wearing turbans like me; others have wigs so like natural hair the difference is difficult to spot. Breast cancer chemotherapy means you lose your hair – not just on the head, but everywhere, including the pubic area, which shocked my friend Lou when it happened to her. I was glad Lou warned me. (When I shower, it is confronting having no hair at all in the pubic area and feels strange.)

I'm lucky because I retained a silvery fuzz atop my head, which my daughter Anne loves caressing just as I used to caress her fluffy head when she was a baby. My John Howard eyebrows and eyelashes thinned much to Mary Jane's delight — her tweezer fingers left unsatisfied for years because I never wear make-up and refused her attempts to beautify my brows. Universal baldness like some poor alopecia sufferers escaped me, whereas my friend Diane said all her hair – head, face, pubic, underarm, and leg – disappeared down the plughole one morning. A very traumatic parting in the shower! Reading or hearing about the experiences of others confirms that everyone's journey is unique but to share stories is helpful and therapeutic. I recall one of my Irish Mum's sayings: 'Forewarned is forearmed.'

The nurses ask me how I have been between treatments and again I discover information I wish I had known before. I have an injection in the stomach to encourage white blood cells. After the injection, I may experience sudden onset of pain in my bones or a severe headache because my bone marrow is expanding. Another drug, Kytril, taken immediately after the session for two days can also cause a severe headache. I recall the shocking headache experienced after the last session and the days of swallowing Panadol with little relief and relive the stomach churning fear that the cancer has attacked my brain. Now I know it was side-effects and ask if becoming a hypochondriac is also a side-effect of chemotherapy? Jo and I share a laugh.

It is time to be unplugged and farewell the chemotherapy nurses with hugs for a Happy New Year. There will be returns for blood tests but hopefully no more toxic potions. Nothing is ever certain once you live with cancer. It is a silent snake, curled ready to strike when you least expect it. I try to forget the conversations I have had today with those coping with a return after some months, or in some cases, years of remission.

A nurse carries my overnight bag while I wheel the faithful IV machine towards the Oncology Wing. This is my ninth admission and I have stayed in almost every room in this corridor. Nurses, cleaning staff, and food attendants smile recognition. Nurse Hue giggles when I announce, 'The Bald and the Beautiful is back.'

Today a wandering dementia patient means a locked corridor. There is an administrative mix-up and the room I've been assigned already has a resident. Holiday rosters must be a nightmare for hospitals – cancer never takes a rest! The glitch sorted has me sharing a room with Sam from Patterson Lakes whom I discover knows Glenice, one of my guardian angels through this life shattering experience. Six degrees of separation again!

Sam and I share stories and tears. A migrant, she is Cypriot and widowed too. Her husband died fifteen years ago. Sam's daughter is in New York on business and her son recently moved out of home to live with a friend. I sense her loneliness. She is seventy-years-old but looks younger. She discovered a lump one night in bed when she leant on her left side. A lumpectomy followed. I explain Breastscreen, found two lumps in my left breast and I needed a total mastectomy. Today, Sam completed chemotherapy session two. Her hair has been falling out in uneven clumps.

'It is getting so hard to arrange my hair and the bald patches look ugly,' she said beneath a perky leather Dutch Boy cap.

'Shave your head, that's what my oncologist advised.'

'I never thought of that – your head looks good.'

'I don't know about looking good but it sure beats waking up with hair in your mouth, or moulting everywhere like a dog. Glenice shaved my head and I'm sure she'd come to your house and shave yours if you asked.'

'Oh, I can get my daughter to do it when she returns, or I'll go to my hairdresser. What a good idea, I'm glad you told me.'

Grateful to pass on useful information just as I have received hints from others, I reflect on the journey. It is a steep learning curve made easier by support and networking. I give Sam my contact details, 'If you need to talk or cry, I'm only as far away as the phone.'

# Three Months with Cancer

*Joan Budd*

I had breast cancer for three months and then it was gone, kaput, banished, exiled, taken away.

My journey starts thirteen years ago when I went for my annual mammogram at the local breast screen clinic. The yearly pilgrimage was necessary because of my family history.

Maternal grandmother: bowel cancer (deceased).

Mother: pancreatic cancer (deceased).

Sister: breast cancer (deceased).

My health survey form could always raise an eyebrow with a sympathetic look that my demise was inevitable. I, however, did not feel this way at all and found it oddly amusing. Don't misunderstand me. I did appreciate their concern and the compassionate attention they afforded me. It was just that I was healthy and confident my body would hold me in good stead for a long time to come.

After completing the said mammogram, a trickle of blood was detected on the transparent device squishing my right breast while the X-ray was taken. I was asked to sit in the waiting room while a room was prepared for an ultrasound. I had never experienced bleeding from the nipples before, although it was a common occurrence to have my mammogram followed by an ultrasound. After the ultrasound was checked I was sent home, assured that all was okay and to follow up with my GP, which I did the following week. She confirmed my mammogram and ultrasound were okay and off I went.

Approximately two months later I woke with a small stain of blood on my nightie. It had secreted from my right breast. I went immediately to my GP who found a small lump in my right breast. Another mammogram confirmed the lump. My body, which I had held in such high esteem, had let me down. Cancer had invaded. Thoughts crowded my mind like traffic.

*If only we had got it earlier.*

*She left it too late.*

Time was of the essence. The specialist surgeon was a busy man. An appointment loomed way into the future. I couldn't wait. Panic had set in. I was definitely not amused. I had cancer, for God's sake! I needed to see the doctor now.

My pleas were heeded and the next week my husband and I were shown into the specialist surgeon's (who I will call Dr C) room on the top floor of our local private hospital. We were scared beyond belief. We had shouldered our torturous news on our own so far, trying to come to terms with my mortality before involving our family.

We left his room an hour later, two totally transformed human beings. My panic had been replaced with calm optimism. The next step was a biopsy to confirm the state of the lump. Benign or malignant. This was performed in the day surgery unit of the hospital. Two days later the specialist confirmed it was malignant. My calm optimism stayed by my side like a close friend.

After a second visit with the specialist surgeon I felt he was my guardian angel. He explained how serious my situation was. He was honest and direct. My right breast would be removed along with several lymph nodes. He would be with me doing his best work and chances for survival were good, he assured me. My body had let me down, not my strength of will. I was ready for the battle ahead and I felt the need to tell my family, my friends – in fact anyone who would listen: I had cancer. I had never felt stronger and I needed to expose my strength for them. I was scared for sure but it did not keep me from my focus to get my life on track and keep it.

I visited a young physiotherapist, Andrew, who had helped me with my lower back pain. 'Andrew, I have breast cancer and I need any help you can give me.' I remembered him telling me how he had helped his mum through her battle with the dreaded disease. I lay on my back on his table and he stood at my feet.

'Imagine you have a large army of tiny soldiers at your feet,' he said. 'They are marching through your legs and body, pushing the cancer to the top of your head where it exits your body in retreat.'

I used these positive thoughts for the three weeks before my operation. My naturopath, Rod, had no miracle elixirs to offer but he did prescribe a collection of herbs I placed under my tongue via a dropper for four days before the surgery. This helped my body to cope with the trauma and anaesthetic. I am forever grateful to him.

\*\*\*

In the early hours of the morning of 'Operation Cancer

Day' I looked at my paired breasts and said goodbye to one. They had served me well. (*Now scram! Get lost! You're fired! Get out of here! You're not an arm or a leg – I don't need you*). I choose one breast with a chance to live another day. For the day ahead and the rest of my life.

When I was settled in my room after the surgery I thought I was free of cancer, although Dr C did not agree with me. I needed a five year term on a prescription medication called Tamoxifen. I called this my insurance policy. Six monthly check ups with Dr C were also required. It took him five years to agree I was cancer free.

I returned home six days after surgery with a drain still intact and with a homecare nurse to visit each day to maintain the drain. Life had never felt so good. The leaves were greener, the sky brighter, ties of family stronger. I embraced life, determined to appreciate it more and never take it for granted. All the clichés when faced with mortality become reality.

My cancer was undetected in the first mammogram, which was of concern for Dr C. On his advice I now attend a private radiology centre for my mammograms. My GP forms part of the surgical team as an observer. I was surprised to see her there. I never questioned why. Maybe there was something to be learned from the circumstances of the detection of the cancer. I will be forever grateful to my caring team, my family and friends, Dr C, and surgical staff, Andrew and his soldiers, Rod and his herbal drops.

Life is beautiful.

# Passage of Grief

*Janette Smith*

The valley, resplendent in golden wattle bloom, hums with the harmony of early morning bustle. Treetop breezes merge with the gurgle of ground waters and the call of the Currawong in flight bears witness to the red-gold edging on the distant horizon. I walk the mountain path I have followed on many mornings and I am lost in memories of a cold spring day on 8th September 1997.

I grew up at the foot of Mt Wellington – since I was a child I have embraced the beauty it brought to my life. The contours and the melody of the mountain have been etched into my memory. When I'm distressed I seek refuge and isolation in the mountain's high places. On the eve before my surgery Rod drove me to the mountain and as the city fell away behind us I watched the sharp patterns of light and shade play across the Organ Pipes. The winding road takes us across the northeast face of the mountain and I wind down the window to gasp as sharp slaps of cold mountain air take my breath away. I'm looking for a place that is high but still sheltered from the south-westerly winds that buffet the southern slopes and the exposed summit.

Through a gap in the trees I see a watery reflection and I ask Rod to pull over so I can explore the possibilities. I part the thick musk and dogwood growth to reveal a mountain stream tumbling over mossy stones. I signal to Rod and begin to push my way up a steep overgrown track alongside the stream. Breathless from the steep climb I find a flat spot high above the road, edged by an immense aged log that is home to numerous ferns and mountain peppers. Before long I hear puffing behind me and Rod hands me the champagne and spreads the blanket. Here, beneath tall eucalypts, watching the day slowly drift into night I pop the cork, make a toast to life and take a swig.

I'm not sharing and Rod watches over me as I struggle with the fear that tears at my soul. Our lovemaking is tender, filled with sorrow for tomorrow I must surrender a part of myself. While darkness closes around us we sit cocooned beneath a blanket, the shared heat of our naked bodies keeping the chill at bay. Surrounded by a silent forest Rod holds me in his arms as I speak my fears in hushed tones, lest a word spoken out of place would hurl me further into the abyss. Finally, as snow starts to fall and our feet begin to turn numb, we navigate a slippery path back to the real world to reluctantly face what has to be done.

September 9 is my mother's birthday. Usually a day of celebration but there will be no celebration today. A chill wind blows as we cross the street and, for the third time in two weeks, enter into the corridors of the hospital. No food or water has passed my lips and my head is pounding. The crowded room is shabby and lifeless. A place of waiting. Grey walls and grey floors enclose a disparate assortment of patients who browse tattered magazines and whisper. My body shakes and my teeth chatter uncontrollably as the flow of tears soak my clothes. I feel violated and exposed until a kind nurse approaches quietly and, without a word, wraps a blanket around my shoulders and leads me away from curious eyes into a claustrophobic, but private room.

How do I feel right now? Numb. I look at Rod. He is staring at a magazine, and for some reason I am aware that he hasn't turned the page for the past hour. I can't stand the waiting any longer; I have an insane craving for the injection that will slide the cold fluid into my veins and take me into the sleep of oblivion.

Three days have passed in a haze of drugs but now the drip has been removed and the state of drug-induced euphoria is rapidly leaving me with the reality that I am not just fighting a physical battle. I drift in and out of sleep as the unchecked pain returns and the drains pull at my flesh with every move. I am hungry but no food will pass through the misery that sticks in my throat. My doctor drops by on his morning round. He tries to make me smile with a hearty bedside manner. It doesn't work. He says that I can take a shower today and remove the dressing. As I lie here waiting for Rod I watch the incessant rain lash the window – the flow of tears has stopped; dry upon my face.

I don't know what I expected, but nothing could prepare me for this. I feel the sensation of the hot water on my skin, the soft lather of the soap – then I pull aside the sodden dressing. A row of metal staples march across my chest and disappear under my left arm. I hear someone screaming. Rod steps into the shower, fully clothed, to catch me as I slide down the wall.

I return home feeling vulnerable and isolated. I am disconnected. My four teenage children drift around me – unsure and hesitant. My family is splintered and struggling to endure the fear of losing me. My husband juggles with running the house and his full-time job and the support of family and friends is crucial to our survival. My mother, who fought her own battle with breast cancer eighteen months earlier, calls in every day trying to encourage me out of bed.

'Life is for living, my love,' she says.

I wish everyone would fuck off and leave me alone. They don't understand. Nobody understands. I visit the surgeon in his rooms and I watch impassively as he removes the thick metal staples from my chest. He is so proud of his neat incision. The man needs glasses – or a reality check. I sit at my window watching the days grow longer and the warmth of the sun awakening new life in my garden. I feel nothing. Day after day while I sit our German Shepherd, Bundi, slips inside and lays his head on my lap. He watches me with puzzled brown eyes, now and again giving a soft whimper. He asks me no questions – I tell him no lies.

Another week passes and another visit to the surgeon. It is an effort to get myself ready to venture out into the world. Just getting out of bed is a struggle. Today when I look down at the sling that cradles my left arm I realise how shabby it is. I hesitate, then remove the sling and reach for my favourite scarf to wrap my wounded arm. I put on a touch of lipstick. As I step outside I stop to look at the Spanish blue bells under the Chinese Elm and the tiny white violets spilling across the steps. I stand for a moment listening to the high pitched call of the Spotted Pardalote, the soothing warmth of the sun touches my back.

My doctor acknowledges the scarf and the lipstick with a knowing smile. A very important milestone has been reached, he assures me while he examines his work. And still he raves on about the wonderful neat scar. I don't have the heart to tell him that while I recognise that the red, puckered slash across my chest may have been administered with great surgical skill, and that he may well have saved my life, I *cannot* appreciate this assault to my body as a piece of art.

It is October now and my birthday is a quiet day. Spring is in full swing and Mum arrives with a terracotta pot brimming with miniature daffodils. We go to the Botanical Gardens and after a gentle stroll we sit with our backs against sun-warmed stone and talk. Usually a reticent person, Mum's uncharacteristic openness both delights and unnerves me.

By November Mum is unwell and spends most of her days in bed. I cook a quiche and walk to her house hoping to entice her out of bed but she won't budge. My stepfather, Arthur, seems distracted and I feel like he is avoiding me. I finally corner him in the garden picking a bowl of raspberries. I am stunned when he gives in to my persistent questions. My mother is dying. She is losing the battle that we thought was done and dusted almost two years ago. As I stand there in the raspberry patch a cloud drifts across the sun and the afternoon darkens.

Christmas Eve, the weather is warm and humid. I am preparing for Christmas Day when Mum calls. She is in terrible pain and alone in the house. Unable to drive since my surgery I run across the bay but when I arrive, hot and exhausted, I am unable to help her. I call the paramedics and we wait in silence, holding hands both knowing that this time she won't be coming home.

Christmas Day is not worth remembering.

Mum has moved from the hospital to palliative care and I am convinced that if I feed her fresh strawberries she will stay with us longer. Family members are sent on missions to seek the best strawberries in the land. My brother, Michael, and my sister, Deborah, return from the mainland to join the rest of us by her bedside. This is the first time that Mum's five children have been together for over twenty years. We reminisce over family photos and as I watch her chatting happily with her children and grandchildren, I dare to hope that perhaps the strawberries have worked.

Mum slips into a coma. Arthur and I sit on either side of her bed and he sings 'The Star of County Down'. He tells me about the time he first saw her almost forty years ago when he rescued her from unwanted attentions at a country dance in Western Victoria. He tells me how they fell in love and eventually she left my father and ran away to join him in Tasmania. While Mum lies between us, perhaps aware of his words, Arthur shares his deepest feelings of love and grief with me, his stepdaughter.

The heat is unbearable today. Bushfires are raging on the southern outskirts of Hobart. Rod encourages me to take a break and walk to Salamanca Place. My head is spinning with the smoky heat. We sit in the shade of the Plane trees and watch the passing crowd. I drink a pint of Guinness. When we return to the hospital my sister, Maureen, tells me that Mum died only moments before. Wednesday, 21 January 1998.

I walk into the cool room and take her hand in mine. I listen to the hum of the ceiling fan and watch the curtains move in the light breeze. I am empty. I become aware of a faint sound and I look up to see Arthur crouched in the shadows of the room. I stand, walk around the bed and kiss the top of his head and leave him alone with his grief.

Maureen and I bathe Mum in scented water. As sisters we are locked in the intimate ritual of cleansing our dead mother. We clothe her in a soft white gown. With an ache in my heart I gently brush her hair. She is at peace, serene and beautiful in death. I rest my lips on her brow and whisper words of love then turn and walk to the door. Here I linger, locked in time and unable to break that invisible cord that has bound us together for forty years. Finally I walk the empty corridor, a passage of loneliness and grief.

Soon after Isobel's death her ashes are returned to her beloved Ireland. On a clear spring day in County Down her cousin, Winifred, puts the urn under her arm and crosses the field. Walking into the woods where they played as children she removes the lid and with a silent prayer scatters the ashes beneath the trees. Ashes to ashes, dust to dust.

It is now fourteen years since I first heard that word 'cancer' directed at me. It still doesn't feel like it is connected to me; there is a sense of it being somebody else's journey. For a long time after Mum's death I struggled to separate her death from the fear of my own. I felt as though I was dwelling in a void. Perhaps in response to this fear, I made the decision to have my other breast removed. It was difficult for my husband to understand why I was taking this action but I was making a deeply personal decision and I walked a lonely road. I returned to work two months after this surgery but I had lost my self-confidence and I was still struggling with depression and self-pity.

Twelve months after the diagnosis of breast cancer, our twenty-four year marriage was struggling and we separated for eight months. During the separation while I was trying to manage full-time work and caring for four teenage children I finally hit rock bottom. I've often heard the saying 'The only place to go when you reach rock bottom is up' and for me that was the catalyst. I began to make life-changing decisions and I followed my dreams, slowly at first, taking small steps in the right direction.

I love nature and bushwalking so I joined a walking club which opened up a world of beautiful experiences in the Tasmanian wilderness. I also had the opportunity to share this love and the experiences with my family and friends. I aspired to attend university but as I had left school at the age of fourteen, and I was committed to full-time work to help support my family, it seemed an impossible dream at the time. However, following eight years of part-time study I finally graduated with an Associated Degree in Arts in 2010 and I'm currently working on a Bachelor of Fine Arts.

My husband and I now live on a six-acre property nestled into the forest on the side of Mt Wellington. In 2010 we came achingly close to losing our second son and once again I had to pick myself up from rock bottom but here, where the views to the southeast go on forever and the rhythm of life is revealed, every day is an inspiration. As I walk the mountain paths I listen to the pulse of the mountain and the harmony of the forest and I hear my mother's words, 'Life is for living, my love.'

# Bower Bird

*Loula S Rodopoulos*

Perched on a cemetery rock poetic pen finds peace
Spins and weaves through village life
To explore mortality it seeks
Across the globe takes flight

Spins and weaves through village life
Poetic pen reflects on the past to pass the day
Across the globe takes flight
A bower bird in word play

Poetic pen reflects on the past to pass the day
Pawns emotions   excites pleasure   nurtures life
Placates the scarred breast
A bower bird in word play
Will it ever rest?

Pawns emotions   excites pleasure   nurtures life
Placates the scarred breast
To explore mortality it seeks
Will it ever rest?
Perched on a cemetery rock poetic pen finds peace

# The Fake One

*Karen Lethlean*

Marjorie and Fred migrated from England to Australia after World War II. They were in search of steady work and maybe better weather than they were used to in England. There wasn't enough room on the immigration paperwork for middle names so the family inserted only first names. In 1952, Majorie, by then in her late forties, was thrilled to discover she was pregnant. Michael, whom she referred to as her 'change of life baby', was to become my husband. His parents used to joke that their son was proof that their new country was more fertile. Even though I wasn't part of his carefree childhood near the shores of Lake Monger, I'd heard stories about those years bathed in the bright sunshine and fresh air of Perth's northern suburbs.

One significant moment in the to and fro that preceded Micheal's marriage was when I sat down with Majorie with family photo albums. I was nervous, but Majorie must have found it difficult to contemplate how quickly Micheal had grown into an adult, and swept aside lingering doubts about his choice of bride.

Among the various snaps were professional studio portraits taken when Micheal had been a child model for Boan's store at the tender age of six. Even back then his good looks and impish grin were evident. My future mother-in-law and I seemed to share a moment that was more about common love than barriers of culture or generations.

For Majorie, parenting a new baby in this conservative time in Australian history when breastfeeding was seriously frowned upon must have been difficult. The fifties mother was told to train her babies onto regulated feeding times only from a bottle. Women who breastfed were regarded as peasants, backward and lacking in the modern sanitation methods necessary for sterilising bottles.

By the time I met Marjorie she had already lost one breast to cancer. Who knows the reasons why? Was it due to not breastfeeding? Or was it an unruly gene? Maybe a restricted war-time diet was another factor? Whatever the reason her preventative choices in the 1970s were extremely limited. The thought of self-examination in the era was all too hideous to contemplate. Women simply didn't touch their own breasts! Her cancer must have been well advanced by the time it was diagnosed.

I try to imagine what might have happened. Maybe she noticed a lump that didn't go away or an unusual discharge or swollen red areas that brought her to the doctors for tests. Just as there was no campaign on public television and in magazines for self-breast examination there was also no such thing as regular mammograms. Women did not go to their doctors if they did notice small breast lumps. More than likely they were patted paternalistically on the head and told to go home and not worry, as it was just part of their menstrual cycles.

And if the lump turned out to be cancer? There was only one option. Surgery. The greatest fear was that a routine biopsy would mean that you woke from anaesthesia with a radical mastectomy. Consult, discuss with or actually consider the patient's feelings – whatever for?

Marjorie's cancer must have been too severe for any treatment other than removal. I still cannot help thinking this was a first rather than a last option back then. Little thought was given to any psychological impact, especially for something that was regarded as insignificant as a breast! Marjorie was given a prosthetic to slip inside everyday brassieres. It wasn't at all realistic and must have been very uncomfortable in summer. I could see the flat pink-beige thing inside some of her lightweight summer blouses. She used to enjoy the silk numbers she had bought on trips to Hong Kong and Singapore. There was no plastic surgery, no insertion of implants. Women like Marjorie were simply told to be strong, to stop any vanity and just get on with life.

*You are just like an Amazonian with a breast removed to make it easier to throw a spear. The diseased part has been chopped away and you will be right, darl.*

*Oh, you say you'd like to swim? Well too bad as the 'falsie' can't get wet. We don't have anything to offer you for that activity; you could, of course, just go without and show your flat no-breast to the world but who would want to see that? You're too old to go swimming now anyway.*

The strongest memory of my in-law's visit to our Melbourne house, after our wedding, was the day Marjorie held out the falsie, wobbling like a skin tone jelly, in her hand.

'Touch it, it's got a nipple.'

Sure enough there was a hard lump off-centre amongst the glutinous mass that looked more like the bean-bags we had at school than anything else. Why she did this I can only imagine. What shock value motivated her to bring out the fake one, push it at me, and make me hold it? Perhaps she wanted to jab at my complacency. Perhaps she had seen me looking. Maybe the show and touch idea was to debunk any myths of complacency in my head. I was shaken to my core.

Little more than a naïve teenager, I must have been agape at touching another woman's – for all intended purposes – breast. What a prudish creature I was back then! With the benefit of hindsight I now think this might have been a strange kind of experiential warning. In her own way Marjorie was trying to tell me the possible outcome of ignorance.

Sure enough by the time I had been married three years to Michael the cancer had again invaded Marjorie's body – her lymph system and liver were taken by the advancing tumours. She was not expected to live very long. We began to actively pursue a compassionate posting back to Western Australia.

'I'll pretend I'm sicker than what I really am,' was her comment to us about facing the officials that came to interview everyone to establish grounds for relocation. Marjorie, Fred, doctors, specialists and other family members were interrogated to assess the likelihood of us being transferred to either the SASR at Swanborne or to Swan Barracks in Perth. With a minimal army population, it was difficult to score Western Australia as a military posting. We just hoped that compassionate grounds would assist.

Marjorie's illness, however, was never an act. I was to witness the vomiting and attempts to cope with the cycles of chemo. Her hair fell out. Again. Once Marjorie showed me her hard swollen torso. 'Feel that,' she said and, sure enough, nestled under her ribcage was something the shape of hard skinned melon.

Once all three of her children were back in Perth, Marjorie made a decision. It was 1980. She told us she no longer wanted to continue with treatment. She couldn't see the point arguing; that doctors were never going to find a cure in her lifetime. Marjorie did not seem to want us to try to convince her otherwise; she'd resigned herself to the forces of fate. She had fought an epic battle, but it was time to concede that this personal war could not be won. She spent time with each of her children and made decisions as to who would inherit the many treasures collected during world travels.

My marriage to Michael did not survive but we had a daughter. Marjorie never met the wonderful granddaughter who seems to have inherited her grandmother's peaches and cream complexion and tall, graceful appearance. But as a token of reverence to Marjorie, we kept the first name only idea alive.

A diamond in white gold heart pendant sits as a symbol of Marjorie's strength and generosity on either my, or our daughter's cancer-free chests, and even if it's not being worn I like to think it still beats with its own memories.

# A Change of Heart and Mind

*Janet Baker*

We all have hopes and dreams and wish to live long and healthy lives, but for many that dream shatters, and a hand is dealt for which we seem ill-prepared.

*Sandra is married to Bill and has four adult children: Will (living in America with his partner Lisa); Dean (living in London with his partner Jamie); Terese (and her partner Chris); and Michael (and his partner Renuka).*

*Sandra is also my sister-in-law and shares with me one of those life-changing times when one's spirit and strength is truly tested.*

## How my journey began

It began with the death of my younger brother, Greg, to lung cancer on 26 May 2005; he left behind his wife Rhonda and three children, Rebecca 21, Amanda 19, and Scott 17. I had also lost my older brother, Malcolm, to bowel cancer on the 11 May 1980; he was 36 and left his wife, Heather, and two young children Sean 3, and Peter nineteen months.

I struggled with the fact that my two siblings had died with the same terrible disease, leaving my youngest brother Garry and me. It left me thinking quite a bit about cancer and its causes. If only I could find out why. I was  constantly told that because they had different cancers the types are not related but I couldn't help but wonder when they both, along with my husband, had worked in a factory handling raw, blue asbestos for at least two years. If these asbestos particles could enter the lungs, then why could they not enter other parts of the body via the skin, or the bloodstream? These thoughts haunted me.

I remember clearly standing at my workstation not long after Greg's death, staring out the window and thinking I too had cancer. I was going through depression, but didn't realise it at the time. I would look at myself in the mirror and think how much I had suddenly aged, how dull and lifeless my eyes seemed to be. They had lost their sparkle – you know that spark of life you see in a person's eyes. I had lost all enjoyment of life, such as gardening, walking my dog, the immense pleasure of my cat's watchful and playful presence, and above all, outings with my family and friends.  It was all ... gone. I felt as though I just existed, but I couldn't understand why.

**Monday 10 April 2006**
I was working at home grooming dogs; I picked up the phone to call a customer and found a message had been left on it. The woman's voice came over very clearly and precisely: 'This is a private message for Sandra Baker from BreastScreen at Liverpool regarding your recent mammogram; please call Helen when you receive this message.'

My heart thumped; my stomach churned. I had been on HRT for thirteen years, which – owing to media reports on safety reports surrounding HRT – I knew was a long time. I had mammograms religiously every two years and had never had a call back for anything. My mind raced. I rang immediately, unable to concentrate on anything else.

Helen – the liaison nurse – told me very kindly that they had found something on the x-rays. 'Please don't panic, these things are usually nothing; probably a cyst or benign lump, but we need to make sure.' She asked if I could come in on Thursday of that week, 13th April (a date I will never forget). 'We do all the testing on the day so there is no going home and wondering what your fate may be. We will do another mammogram and if we aren't satisfied with the outcome, then we do an ultrasound; and then, if necessary, a fine needle biopsy so you have a result there and then.' Helen asked me to come in at 9.00 am and to expect to be there for two to four hours. I was sick in the stomach and felt straight away this was not good.

When I told my husband, he told me not to worry, it would be nothing. I then told Michael and Terese as they arrived home from work. They all told me not to worry, it would be nothing; people are called in for these things all the time only to be told everything is okay. I calmed down considerably and began telling myself it *would* be okay.

**Thursday 13 April: The Clinic**
By the time my husband and I arrived at the clinic, I was not worried at all – well, maybe a little doubtful. Reluctantly, he dropped me off after I assured him I would be fine.

I sat in my gown looking around at the other women in the clinic, wondering if we were all going to be all right; or would someone's world be plunged into dire uncertainty. As each one went in with fingers crossed, they returned shortly afterwards with a big smile and the thumbs up; we all breathed a little easier. Sheer relief was in their eyes and on their faces. I was the last to go in and now I know why. I think they keep the doubtful ones until last to avoid upsetting others unnecessarily.

I walked into the x-ray room and my films were up on the board. As soon as I looked at them I knew it wasn't good. The young radiographer looked at me and said, 'It may just be a cyst.'

I replied, 'I don't think so.'

She said she would do another mammogram for the doctor to have a look at. This was done, and the doctor then came in and told me they needed to do an ultrasound to confirm their suspicions.

I lay on the bed and watched the progress on the screen. I saw the dark lump in my breast and said to the radiographer, 'That's not good, is it?'

She replied, 'I don't think so.'

She asked me to lift my arm to examine my armpit. Surges of overwhelming dread engulfed me. I hadn't even thought about lymph nodes being involved. I saw straight away the telltale dark patch, and again uttered my previous words, 'That's not good, is it?'

Her reply: 'No it isn't.'

*That's it, I'm dead! Once it's in the lymph nodes you've had it.* The radiographer told me she had to confer with the doctor and that I may have to have a fine needle biopsy. I lay there crying. *I'm dying; how could I have not known but, maybe I did.* How many times had I thought this?

All I could think of was my husband, Billy, and how was he going to cope without me? Who would look after him? How would my children cope? The older two would be all right as they were both settled, and had lived overseas for at least thirteen years. They have lives without their parents being involved so I knew they would cope reasonably well. The younger two were still living at home and I felt they depended on me.

My animals, they wouldn't understand why I had gone suddenly. My dog Darcy loved his daily walks. Who would do this? My husband couldn't due to a permanent work injury.

I wasn't ready to die; I didn't want to leave my family and friends. Thoughts of everyone began flashing through my mind. Would I get to see enough of them before the end? How could this be happening to me? It's always someone else. Now I know how they must have felt; no other person's suffering prepares you for your own.

The fine needle biopsy was done. I didn't even find it painful, just uncomfortable; perhaps shock dulls all. The result was positive for cancer cells in the breast and armpit.

I couldn't stop crying and apologised to everyone. I felt like such a baby. Why couldn't I be brave? It was more about the thought of leaving everyone that upset me, not the dying. The staff were wonderful. They tried to cheer me up, and even had me smiling. I dressed and Helen, the liaison nurse, came in with the doctor to speak with me. They told me what they thought my treatment might involve: surgery, chemotherapy and possibly radiation. I was given choices of doctors recommended by the clinic or I could search out my own surgeon, along with my GP's advice.

Helen shared with me her own breast cancer experience. Her circumstances were almost identical to mine, and yet, here she was sixteen years later and still healthy.

I left the clinic feeling numb and went out to meet my husband. It was raining, which somehow seemed appropriate. He was light-hearted when he asked how it went. All I could say was, 'It's not very good.' I still remember the stunned look on his face. Then, I told him what had happened. I also recall telling him about a conversation I had with my sister-in-law Jan, in January 2006, prior to my finding out about the breast cancer. It went something like this:

Jan had rung me to ask if everything was okay with me. Was I feeling well and was everyone else in the family all right? I replied that all was okay as far as I knew. Jan then went on to tell me about some recurring dreams she had been having about me; they were bothering her and she had felt an urgency to ring and let me know.

She dreamt that my father visited her all dressed in white and his message was to tell me everything would be all right. She also had two dreams about my mother. In the first, my mother was dressed in an overcoat with large round buttons. My mother's message was the same, to tell Sandra everything will be all right. In the second dream, my mother was in a group photo with names listed underneath. One name was circled 'White'.

She indicated that Sandra should be told – Jan had to tell me.

The only thing I could think of that might relate to something being, or going, wrong was that I would be travelling to America in the August with my daughter Terri to visit my son Will, and Lisa, who live in San Francisco. This was to be my first plane trip, and I was very worried about taking it. I had always been terrified of flying, but had always wanted to visit them. So, I concluded that this was what the message was about; it was fine to fly.

Jan and I discussed the dreams at length, and she told me she was unsure that the message was about flying. In any case, she said, 'You will know when it happens.' We decided to keep this to ourselves to wait to see what eventuated, if anything.

I didn't think about that conversation again until travelling home that day. After relating the story to Billy, he said, 'That is eerie; it gives me goosebumps. But, it's a good sign, and I don't usually believe in anything like that. It really makes you think.' I too decided it was a very positive message to take on board. (I was to recall it almost every day for the next two years. I still think of it today whenever the dark, cancer thoughts enter my mind, which is often.)

**Home**
I walked into my home and just stood, unsure what to do. I felt different. Everything seemed normal but, I was now *different*; would I ever feel like me again?

I told my son and daughter when they came home and rang my other two sons and other family members as soon as I could. Although everyone was shaken, they all felt that I would be okay. This was very comforting, even though I was still afraid.

I recall lying in bed that night, so afraid ... and in utter disbelief. *I was going to die!* I wanted to fall asleep and find when I awoke in the morning it had been a dream. I was crying and Billy reached over and held me close. I can't begin to tell you how comforting that was. You don't realise how much you need another human's touch, especially in times of crisis. The strange thing was I had been lying there wishing my mother were still here to comfort me.

Soon thereafter, I chose one of the doctors from the hospital's list and rang for an appointment.

Most Sunday mornings we'd take our dog Darcy to Kurnell and walk along the beach. This time Michael, Renuka, and Terese came with us. It was a beautiful day and good to all be together but, I couldn't enjoy it. I felt alone; as if I were an island, isolated; some invisible observer of another world I was unable to be part of, or enjoy. *Their lives are really still the same. They can go to sleep at night and feel normal; I couldn't feel normal; I didn't feel like I did five days ago.* I was not to shake that feeling for a long, long time.

My mind went into overdrive. What did I do wrong? Somehow I did this to myself. Never mind the fact that I was never able to find a definite reason for my elder brother Malcolm's cancer. I knew the cause of Greg's cancer: smoking combined with the effects of asbestos. That, at least, made sense to me. What was the cause of mine ... possibly HRT but what else? There had to be other factors: I was overweight at 87kg and insulin resistant. I had suffered for sixteen years with chronic diarrhoea with no known cause, even after having regular colonoscopies. My doctors had no answers. I didn't have any of the known diseases associated with this symptom. It had become so bad I loathed leaving the house, let alone go on a special outing. That was usually out of the question unless I had easy access to a toilet.

I told myself not another piece of rubbish would pass my lips. No more Coca Cola, lollies, chocolate, dairy, fat or anything I thought was suspicious. I began researching: books, the internet, and talking to anyone who would listen and had an opinion. I haunted my local health store. The girls there were great and helped me endlessly. Any information they came across they passed on to me, while at the same time always being positive about everything. I'm sure my family suffered as I would constantly ask them not to eat, or drink this or that. 'Please don't use deodorant; don't put that on your hair; and whatever you do don't paint your nails or use false nails; it will kill you.' They humoured me and tried to avoid upsetting me. Even in the supermarket, I spent hours going over ingredients' labels, and scowling at the contents of people's trolleys. I had to restrain myself from telling them to put most of the products they had selected back on the shelves, and never to touch them.

I spent a small fortune on vitamins and books, and I spoke at length to my daughter's singing teacher. She had always been into health products and now owned a health food store. She was able to put me onto a retired oncologist who had some success treating cancer with special diets. This doctor had worked overseas in an 'alternative' cancer hospital. I went to see her at her home in Balmain and she gave me very good advice along with a diet, foods to avoid, and certain vitamins to take. I followed her advice to the letter – except for the coffee enemas. *That*, I could not do by myself.

Coffee enemas utilise coffee and purified water (under specific guidelines) for the purpose of cleansing the blood and detoxifying the liver; however, it is best to seek appropriate and qualified guidance in their use.

### The Surgeon's Visit

He was wonderful.

I met with him two weeks after being diagnosed. He told me he was unable to detect my lump from physical examination as it was very deep against the chest wall. My GP had also examined me and could not feel the lump, and also said he would never have known I had breast cancer simply from that examination; I was lucky I had regular mammograms.

My surgeon thought I may not have to have chemo; maybe just the radiation. I had wanted to have a mastectomy because I wanted to get rid of it. My surgeon talked me out of it, saying this wasn't necessary in my case. He would operate and make sure he had taken enough of a margin to be safe and I would still have my breast. He was sure I would feel a lot better in myself by doing this as the chemo and radiation were enough to deal with. He told me I would be okay and that was very important to me. After such a positive discussion, Billy and I came out of his surgery feeling elated, and for the first time I felt that I might get through this and *live*. I think I floated all the way home.

The next six weeks went by in a daze. I was unable to work and had a friend come in and take over the dog grooming for me.

My son Dean flew in from London. His resolve and unwavering support helped restore my faith in my ability to make some difficult choices. He took control and organised things while reinforcing, 'You'll be okay, and you will get through this.' Will and Lisa wanted to fly over as well. But, after much consideration, we talked Will out of it because really, there was nothing he could do and we felt it would be better to save the flight for a later time when we might need him, or when I was feeling better and able to enjoy his visit.

**Pre-operation**
The day before the operation, I went to the Nuclear Medicine clinic for the dye and fine wire to be inserted into my breast. This was done without any anaesthetic. I was forewarned it would be extremely painful and I may faint – as many patients do.

The nurse stood beside me and told me to squeeze his hand as hard as I wanted. I don't know if I was still in some sort of shock, but I was able to tolerate it without any tears or grimacing. I simply told myself it had to be done and it would be over quickly.

It was a sharp, hot, stomach churning, sickening pain, and looking back, I don't think I would like to have it again.

**Tuesday 23 May: The Operation**
My operation was on schedule.

While lying on the bed waiting for my turn, I had

an extraordinary experience. I dreamt that Our Lady came and visited me. She stood at the bottom of my bed, between mine and the next bed. Lying in the next bed was Martina, the sister of my former daughter-in-law's mother. (Martina lived in Ireland and was going through ovarian cancer.) Our Lady told us that we would both be all right. There was a brilliant light radiating from her as she looked down upon us. I felt it was a healing light; it was as if I could feel it going through my body. It was so comforting.

I had the lumpectomy and fifteen lymph nodes removed. We knew the sentinel node was involved because it had shown up on the ultrasound, but we didn't know if it had spread to any others. The biopsy showed that all the other nodes were clear as well as the tissue surrounding the tumour. That was a big plus. My surgeon was very happy with the results and again, he thought, I may escape chemo – how wonderful.

I felt strangely elated during my hospital stay; I think I was on some sort of high from the dream or the anaesthetic, or both. I was to have many very spiritual experiences along this journey.

**Treatment strategy**
Once home, I needed a follow-up appointment to meet with my oncologist in June. It was all very surreal because I didn't feel ill.

While waiting in the cancer clinic at Campbelltown Hospital, the liaison nurse came to speak with me as she had done when I was in hospital. She informed me that at any time I felt uncomfortable with any of the doctors,

I was welcome to ask to see someone else. I said that I knew the doctor I was about to see was the same doctor who had treated my late brother, but that I would feel more comfortable, in this situation, if I could see a female doctor. It was arranged there and then with no fuss. I'm so glad I did.

(I felt I had a very good relationship with my oncologist and all the doctors and registrars who treated me; as well as my GP whom I have known for thirty years.)

The first meeting went well and I was given all the information about my expected treatment; however, it was still undecided about the necessity for chemo.

There was a meeting between all the oncologists, the radiotherapy oncologist, and my surgeon, to discuss my best options. The decision was made; I was to have chemo, much to my disappointment. They all felt it was much safer to do this because of the lymph node involvement.

**Researching treatment options**
This is where my own research almost brought me undone.

I had read many times about the dangers of chemo and what it could do. I had also been told by the oncologist about some *possible* side-effects such as heart attack during treatment, a weakening of the heart, and leukaemia down the track. I began to think the cure was worse than the disease and how could this possibly cure me. Natural alternatives were the way to go as far as I could see. How could you heal your body by injecting it with poison?

I had been speaking, by phone, to a young woman who had breast cancer with lymph node involvement and how she had decided to have the operation, but forgo the chemo and radiation. We talked for many hours about alternative medicine, and she and her husband had done an enormous amount of research. She was going to a national laboratory in Sydney every month to have her blood and markers monitored as well as her organs and her nutrition. This was costly and not something I could afford to do.

I was dead set against chemo, and the day before my treatment began, I decided not to do it.

Billy and I were on our way to see our GP, and I told Billy I really didn't want to go ahead with it. He was upset and felt I should do it, but he said it was my choice and he would support whatever I wanted to do.

In my doctor's surgery, I told him of my decision. He was appalled and told me that if I didn't go ahead with it he would be gravely concerned for my life. He told me of a case he knew of where the person had decided to try alternative medicine and was now fighting for their life because the cancer had spread to their liver and bones; they were now having chemo ... but, it was probably too late. I never did ask what happened.

**Thursday 6 July: A change of mind**
My doctor's story resonated deeply and ... yes! I did change my mind. I went ahead with the chemotherapy.

I remember going to my first session. I was to have it every three weeks for three months, then a different course for the following three months. I was told that with the first drug treatment (Dolasetron and Dexamethasone)

I would lose my hair and I would feel quite ill – and possibly have nausea and vomiting as well. I was to stay away from anyone who had an illness, avoid shopping centres, and anywhere there was a large gathering of people. This was to avoid picking up any germs because my immune system would be very low. I had to constantly monitor my temperature and if it changed, even slightly, I was to go straight to the hospital. I was given a red card to show on arrival, which stated my condition to the staff – scary stuff. I also had to avoid being in the sun because the chemo would cause me to sunburn very quickly. I was given Phenergan to help reduce any reaction to the chemicals. I slept through the session.

After leaving the hospital later that afternoon, I was surprised to be feeling all right, just tired. This lasted for two days but then it hit me – the worst feeling of nausea I have ever known. At least I wasn't vomiting; I hate vomiting and always fight it for as long as possible. Had I been susceptible to vomiting I wouldn't have fared as well as I did during the treatments.

I wanted to lie down and die. It's very hard to explain just how bad you feel, but it is as though you are bordering on the edge of death. Aside from the constant nausea, feeling totally exhausted, and struggling to get through each day, I felt as though I was in a deep, black hole, trying to get back out, but couldn't. I just wanted to give up. I've been told by the nurses that you are given enough of the chemicals to kill off all the cells in your body without actually killing you; that's how they kill off the cancer cells. Is it any wonder you are so susceptible to picking up germs and feel so gravely ill?

The miracle of all this is that for around five to seven days you feel you are at death's door and then you begin to recover. The nausea is continuous, but nowhere near as bad as that first week. You have two weeks' reprieve and before you know it you are back again for the next treatment. After each session I really didn't think I could go on or that I would make it to the next one.

Without my family I don't know how I would have made it through. Every time I would say I wasn't going on with it, Billy and Michael would come in and talk with me. They would point out how far I had come, even after the first time. They would say something like, 'One down, only five more to go and in a few days you will start to feel better again; you only have to get through this week.'

Clarity dawned. I needed someone to constantly point this out to me. The chemo messes with your head badly, and you can't think, concentrate, or make decisions; you need to see some rays of light emerging through a thickening fog. Your cognitive function goes out the window – hence the term 'chemo brain'; it really is a condition.

I had also lost a lot of weight, which was a concern for everyone around me. It was partly due to my changed diet, but you also lose your appetite. I would feel hungry then not know what I wanted to eat. I'd think of a food and within minutes, even seconds, no longer feel like it. I mostly felt like salty things – especially Asian type soups. (Such was my desire for Asian cooking – and I don't know how I did it feeling so ill – I took a two day Chinese cooking course at the community college.)

### Side-effects

Yes – my hair! I began to think I was going to be lucky and my hair would not fall out. It had been three weeks and it was still intact. I went in for my next appointment and they all assured me that *it would fall out*. I remember one night going to bed and my head was sore all over. I thought then that I would wake up in the morning with no hair, but I still had it; none on the pillow.

After walking the dog, I came back and showered. As soon as I ducked under the water I knew it *was* going to come out; and so it did – in handfuls. I dried and dressed and suddenly picked up my dog clippers (with a number ten shaving blade) and clipped it all off; I didn't want bald patches and bits of hair constantly falling everywhere.

I looked in the mirror: *this is it*! All I can say is that having no hair does have its advantages: no more worrying about how your hair looks and having to look after it. Wash and go – how easy. It's so cool in summer, but surprisingly cold in winter. You just don't realise how warm your hair keeps you; a beanie is crucial in winter.

One of the best experiences I had was walking in gentle rain without a hat. It felt like little bubbles bursting on my head; a fizzy feeling. I was a happy, carefree child walking through the bush in the rain – *with no hair*.

### Revelations

There are many positives when you go through cancer and its treatment. You meet the most amazing people, and it makes you very humble indeed. I do think you begin to take a lot more notice of other people's circumstances. You realise how fortunate you are to be alive, and that the things you are suffering are nothing compared to what so many others have to endure. You really do have to try very hard to overcome negative thoughts that make you feel so bad and try to only think about the good things of life.

It's a mind game.

For some strange reason, your mind wants to take you to 'the depths of despair'. It's almost as if you have two minds: one can be so destructive in its thinking; and the other, so hopeful and full of good thoughts. I know most of this was caused by the chemicals, and it was a constant battle not to let myself succumb. I'm sure many people do just that – particularly after the chemo. It would scare the hell out of me, which was probably good, because then I would say to myself, *Oh no, don't think this way, I'm not ready to go yet, there are too many things I want to see and do before I go.* It would be very easy to give in and decide to end it there and then; it's much harder to fight it.

**Return to the spiritual**

I began going to church again after a ten-year absence. A good friend, Clare McManus, encouraged and helped me do this. I would sit in church and the priest, Father Sarkis, would read the Homily – I could swear he wrote it just for me. I would feel that Jesus was sitting beside or in front of me. I felt him near; just sitting, silently, with me. I felt such joy and elation as if I were blessed. I would also feel that my brothers and parents were with me all the time. I could see my parents and the message they gave to Jan; it would constantly jump before my eyes and I would feel it going through my body.

Everyone at Our Lady Help of Christians was wonderful to me. I was very lucky to have their friendship, prayers, and concern. I was not the only one going through the torment of this insidious disease. I knew of others in our parish, in particular Geraldine, who was young and with three young children to care for (one of whom was only seven-months-old); and Sue, who had been battling ovarian cancer four years previously and was in remission. (Sadly, Sue passed away in 2010; she had lived with cancer for around six years.) We had many chats together about the positive effect faith could have on you.

One Saturday, standing at my local butcher's counter, I was tapped on the shoulder. A lovely voice said, 'Do you mind if I ask, are you going through chemotherapy'? I replied that I was. This beautiful young woman then pointed to her lovely curly hair and said, 'This came from having chemo twelve months ago.' She was gorgeous, around twenty-two-years-old and newly married. She introduced herself and told me her story. Her words were so encouraging. I couldn't believe that she could be so lovely and happy after all she had gone through. She then told me that she had found out that week that her cancer had come back. Her attitude to it was amazing. She only thinks of the future and how she and her husband had made plans for their children and home. 'Nothing is going to stop me,' she said. We wished each other well and I thought I would never see her again – but, I did.

I was talking to my neighbour about her son who had bowel cancer at nineteen-years and how it had returned; he was twenty-six-years old at the time. (He unfortunately passed away in 2010.) I told her of the young woman and my neighbour then told me she knew this girl's parents. We arranged to meet with them at my neighbour's home.

I was so sad to see her with no beautiful curls but, she still had her wonderful attitude and big smile. She told me the curls will come back after the treatment. I know she had many 'battles for her life' during this second bout of treatment, and many times had to be isolated; but, she is such a fighter and inspiration to everyone who knows her.

These are just a few of the most amazing people you meet, and they make such an impact on others' lives.

**Sunday 26 November**
Ten days away from finishing my chemo I suffered a setback.

Coming out of the laundry, barefoot, I stepped straight onto a ball, which my dog had conveniently left there. I had no hope and went down like a sack of potatoes. The sudden and excruciating intensity of the twist made me scream as the pain tore through my foot. I thought it had snapped! I had never felt pain like it before. I thought the wire procedure was bad enough, but for *this*, I was not prepared.

Billy took me to the hospital thinking it was badly sprained. I couldn't put my foot to the floor. I was x-rayed but the doctor couldn't find a break in it. He simply told me to come back if it didn't get any better.

**Tuesday 5 December**
The day finally came for my last round of chemo.

I arrived at the hospital and needed a wheelchair. I couldn't manage the crutches the hospital had given me.

The nurses, in the clinic, were very concerned when they saw how swollen my foot was. I told them what had happened and they went to get my oncologist. She was horrified, and was sure it was broken. She immediately went to the emergency unit and retrieved the x-rays, which showed that my foot *was* fractured in two places. (Apparently, the previous doctor I saw, who didn't spot the fractures, was not the specialist who reads the x-rays. That specialist knew it was broken when he came in and saw the films – the day *after* I had been in the ED; however, nobody, at the time, thought to ring and tell me.)

I was then sent to an orthopaedic surgeon who said he would leave it alone because it had been too long to do anything and the fractures would heal well enough by themselves. I had to stay off my foot but try to move it around when lying in bed to stop it stiffening up. I did this and it did heal really well.

But, it was a terrible time lying there in pain from my foot and the chemo. (The drug, Paclitaxel, used for my second round of treatment was different, which would not make me feel as sick, but it would give me pain instead.) The pain began mainly in my legs and stomach and is very hard to describe; almost like an aching, but more painful. I was given Endone to cope with this and thanked God every day for the invention of drugs – which I hated taking.

**Final Radiation**
Again, I didn't want to have it. Radiation also has its side-effects, such as possibly causing cancer down the track; *this* I tried not to think about.

I was fortunate though to be given the name of a wonderful woman, Diane Cruise, who helped me through the ray treatment without too much burning. She developed a cream, powder and oils to help prevent radiation burns. The radiation treatment lasted six weeks. (Five days each week, except on the alternate weeks I had the Friday off so that the machine could be serviced.) It was at least pain free. I would come home and apply her products as directed. And, you cannot imagine how tired the radiation makes you feel. You really have to rest every day.

Everything went fine until one weekend, when my daughter was moving out of home. I was so busy that I didn't put on any of the products, thinking it would be all right for two days. I was wrong! What I failed to realise was the fact that the radiation continues to burn even when you are not having the actual treatment; this also happens for some weeks after you complete the course. I did end up with a small burn under my breast, but kept using Diane's products and it quickly cleared up. The nurses were amazed at how good my skin was while using this treatment.

**The light at the end of the tunnel**
Finally, it was all over. I had made it. Then Will and Lisa arrived from America, which lifted my spirit immensely.

I would need regular monthly check-ups, then three-monthly, six-monthly, and lastly at twelve-monthly intervals over the next five years. The only hiccup was the hormone drugs the doctors wanted me on after I finished all my treatment. I couldn't tolerate them. They made me so depressed and I couldn't stand feeling that way, so I haven't been on anything since. My GP and the oncologists aren't happy about it, but realise my mental state is more important.

My constant reminder is lymphoedema in my left arm. This has prevented me from working because you are not to lift, hold, pull or push anything over two kilograms. Also, scratches and cuts may be serious if infected. I need to wear a pressure sleeve and glove twenty-four hours a day to keep the lymph fluid moving, to prevent a build up in my arm. This is used together with lymphatic drainage, which I perform on my arm and body every day. It is a nuisance having to do this, but it is a small price to pay for being alive and well.

By the way, my five years are up in April 2012.

So far, so good.

### A change of heart

I try to enjoy and live each day the best I can. I've tried doing things I would never have done before such as snorkelling (what an amazing experience); painting, which is something Jan has tried to get me to do for years; line dancing; and Tai Chi (both for balance, mind and exercise). I totally enjoy them all and am always willing to try something new if it interests me.

I'm back to my gardening and still enjoying spiritual moments; I feel you are never closer to God than being out enjoying nature.

We sold our family home in St Helens Park and moved to a quieter life on the mid-north coast. I still have my moments, but overall am enjoying life up here. And, I *am* me again! I'm so happy.

I have more compassion and understanding for people and their differing circumstances, and I love to be able to offer help to anyone in need. It may be a chat, sitting and listening to how they are feeling, or running an errand. Many elderly people in this area are lonely and unwell and it is a joy to be able to do the simplest thing for them.

Most people like to talk to someone; loneliness can make some so unhappy. For someone to reach out and touch you when you are ill makes you feel safe, loved and cared for; that you belong, are not an island; and are not alone.

*** 

*Sandra's story is one of many. I admire her strength, courage, openness and willingness to share her journey with me. Knowing someone for so many years doesn't mean we really know them. It is only in times such as these that close relationships, friendships and bonds are either brought closer together or broken. At some time in our lives we all need that thread of support; it can be a lifeline. Sandra clung to those threads, however fragile and vulnerable she may have been and came through the other side, enlightened.*

# Going Grey

*Dominique Davidson*

Hairdressers always told me that I had locks of outstanding quality. My hair was like my maternal grandmother's: thick, wavy and dark brown with red fire scattered throughout. It was my shining glory.

I saw the first ones when I was twenty-three. To my eye, the grey hairs stood out like warts on an appendage. Unlike the warts, I was able to pluck them out. This I did until there were too many and I succumbed to the security of hair dye.

Apparently *going grey* is an inherited characteristic. My paternal grandmother and her sister went grey before they were thirty. I was not pleased. Why did I have to inherit this? Was it not enough that I did not inherit the long legs, the blue eyes, or the height? Instead, I am five foot nothing, had fat thighs, a long second toe and premature greyness. Meanwhile my brother is tall, blond and blue-eyed. He did have the longer second toe though, and in later years went bald, but that is another story.

I started dying my hair before my first marriage ended, so I must have been about twenty-seven. My first foray into hair dye was as close to my natural colour as I could find; I think it was Clairol Nice 'n Easy, Natural Dark Brown. After the divorce, I went black. I was wearing it in a very chic bob and I thought I looked pretty good, even with the fat legs. My hair grew so fast that I had to dye it every three weeks. It was such a drag. But if I didn't, the *stripe* appeared. Not a good look. The only way to maintain it and my bank balance was to alternate between Cherie, hairdresser extraordinaire, and whatever bathroom I happened to be frequenting. One time, I remember dying it on holidays in New Zealand. I was so vain.

My beauty regime also included extensive waxing. Cherie had a passion for waxing. She was also very talented at it. No blood, no skin loss and a minimal number of ingrown hairs. What girl doesn't appreciate that! A visit to Cherie's was one of the luxuries of my life. I always emerged quaffed and smooth.

I was five weeks and five days post wax. I only had two days to go. It is such a difficult time. You long to bring out the wax strips, but deny yourself. The hairs have emerged again and the occasional ingrown hair has developed into a little pustule that you cannot help but attack, by squeezing and pulling out the offending ingrown hair with the tweezers. I was thirty-nine and three hundred and forty-four days old and at this stage in the waxing/dyeing cycle when I noticed a lump under my arm. *Not good*, I thought. It is either a very large ingrown hair or something very serious.

I waited another two days before going to the doctor. I wanted to keep my appointment with Cherie. I was not going to have a hairy armpit needled. A girl has some pride, you know.

\*\*\*

'Thank God you have Private Health Insurance,' my doctor told me. I was able to get a Fine Needle Aspiration that very same day.

My underarm was beautifully smooth.

They stuck a needle into my lump and aspirated some cells out of it. At thirty-nine and three hundred and forty-seven days old I was told that the pathological diagnosis was *Metastatic Adenocarcinoma*. I had cancer and they didn't know where the original or primary cancer was.

After scans of my body they found that the primary cancer was in my breast and the malignant growth extended to the chest wall. This sort of presentation had very poor prognosis. *Happy Birthday*. On my fortieth birthday I had a double mastectomy with a bilateral axillary lymphadenectomy, which meant I had both my breasts removed and all my lymph nodes under my arms taken out. Both physically and mentally I was a fucking mess.

That was not the end of it. Oh no. As I had not *reproduced*, they suggested that some of my ovary could be removed, just in case I ever wanted to have children. Were they fucking kidding? I was forty-years-old with Stage 3 breast cancer and they were concerned with conserving my reproductive ability? Politely as I could, I declined.

'No thank you.'

\*\*\*

I required both chemotherapy and radiotherapy as part of my treatment. This was because of the Stage 3 nature of my cancer and the fact that the invader extended to the chest wall. To anyone who experiences anything like this, all I can say is that I empathise. I found the experience to be debilitating both mentally and physically. I felt totally betrayed by my body.

This experience has not made me a better person. It has not made me love my life. It has not made me look for every positive in my day. There is no God. I cannot express how it feels to have the coldness of the chemotherapy entering your veins and invading your body. How it makes you puke and puke and puke until you think that you will die from puking.

*** 

The therapy is so much worse than the surgery.

*** 

Now that I have so very little hair, and don't bother to dye it anymore, I ponder: what the hell is wrong with grey hair? Throughout my twenties and thirties, I had devoted so much time, energy and money to avoiding going grey. I would give anything now to have a full head of grey hair and no cancer.

I turned forty-one last week. I shouted myself a luxurious wig of dark red hair complete with bangs to hide my wrinkled forehead. It looks incongruous with my thin wizened body, but less hideous than the white, sparse wisps of hair that now grow on my head. The wig certainly looks less hideous than the black woollen beanie that I had taken to wearing.

*** 

I had my follow up scan yesterday. Tomorrow, I'm going to see Cherie and get my nails done.

# The Good Breast

*Gaylene Carbis*
*for Lynette Owen*

This is benign
no big deal. some
abnormal
fibrous tissue.
the Doctor with the many degrees
has said: Have it out.
Get it removed.
And he makes an appointment
for this *simple* operation.

the doctors we see are always
male and have an awesome authority.
their methods are incisive.
he recommends a straightforward
surgical procedure:
I'm in and out quickly.
he's straight to the point, says:
It's not the big C. Nevertheless,
why muck around?
He books me in.

his prescriptions, like sex,
are so purposeful, bent on

instant gratification.
men of medicine seek solutions,
and need results. they
make their meanings,
derive a kind of pleasure from their power
over other people's pain.
his professionalism sits in my stomach,
trivialising the texture of this
specifically female experience.

it comes back to me, how I
make conversation.
I smile, laugh, flirt,
submit like a good girl.
I ask, as though it is my only concern:
how long will I not be able
to swim or dance?
I can't bear for a single day of summer
to be taken from me.

next week,
a cut in my breast.
from these
smooth white breasts
they will remove
a part of me.
my skin forever marked,
a slight scar, a thin line,
the same place on both sides.

it's impossible to breathe in a
body that is not your own.

my father's mother,
my father's sisters,
suffered in silence.
I am the child of cancer.
my father urges me to be careful:
all they refused, you are taking
on, you are
confronting from both sides, those
predecessors: it's a great burden
for your back,
no wonder your breast is heavy.

the women of his family
are within me,
insisting on acknowledgement.
they call attention to inescapable fates.
they tell me to take heed,
to take care,
to remember they
are here,
but when the mind obliterates,
the body begins to murmur.

its flow, its energy, its femaleness
is taken for granted,
and female's ways
are slow and sensual.
no man, no expert can
penetrate beneath;
emotional depth eludes his
training.
healing is in the scalpel, the

knife, the needle.

I don't trust them.
I turn to a nurturing woman:
the earth-mother,
unknown and unacknowledged,
is calling:
the wise woman recognises.
she listens for
layers deeper than tissue.
I lie on her table
and give myself over.

she is asking
for a deeper knowledge,
steeped in ancient wisdom.
she knows my fear,
has felt it and knows the
frustration and fear, the rage beneath.
she is beside me, urging gently:
feel. follow the breath.
focus. feel. breathe into the fear.
let go of the mind. feel your fear.

the women in my father's family,
my aunts, my grandmother,
gather around,
urging me not to follow
in their footsteps.
I follow my breath,
I face my fear.
with my friend

holding my hand
all the way through
her hand on my chest,
my breast. so soothing.

I return to the doctor.
back to see if there are
any other developments
but there's nothing.
I can't find it, he says.
it's gone. disappeared.
he's puzzled, perplexed:
I don't understand.
I do up my blouse. my breasts
are milky and warm and full,
though I'll never be a mother.

we are all mothers
all searching for
our own good breast.
I'm practically blooming
with it. I try to tell him
but as soon as I begin
I see he's sceptical
so I stop. I'm healed.
I walk away whole.
I head out of the hospital,
smiling at everyone
I pass along the way.

everyone.

# The Best of all Possible Cancers

*Teri Merlyn*

I can't say it was a shock when a lump appeared under my fingers during a cursory, half automatic-self-examination, half comforting self-caress. My life was in one of the periodic, vertiginous spirals that summon slapstick filmic and ironic literary euphemisms, such as *The Perils of Pauline* and *Candide*.[1] So, when I was packed off for a biopsy, the result of which was back within sixteen hours, and a peremptory summons came from the GP, I wasn't surprised that the outcome was positive either.

*Hell!* I thought. *Okay! So? What more do* You *have in store for me then?*

It is so much easier to imagine some supernatural intervention as contemplating the random cruelty of such events only serves to enhance one's existential vertigo. Lacking the religious gene myself,[2] childhood exposure to my mother's religiosity still sees Biblical quotes bubbling up at moments of stress.

---

1. At this time I was homeless, having failed to find a new rental by the time notice had expired on my residence of three years and, though a level above couch surfing, at 62 that was pretty stressful. Plus I was engaged in frighteningly spiralling email arguments with both my brother and daughter, who were expressing their concern at my situation in punitive terms. Never, never argue via email!

2. Recent research has identified a gene for profound religious experience.

This time it was the ironic, 'God loves those most whom He tests the most.' *Oh, I see! So You Love Me! That's what this is all about?*

In actuality, my Existential-Libertarian ethos recognises that Fortune can be miraculous, endow all manner of goods, but is also wantonly cruel, and in my life these extremes come in equal measure. So, there I was, hard up against mortality at a time that would already test many mortal's grip on sanity. It is not that Death is an unusual topic of consideration for me. Indeed, my tumultuous state of being was inculcated at the breast and I had early on recognised only two certainties:

One: I was alive.

Two: one day I'd be dead.

Even as a child, I was more curious why people carried on so about others dying than distressed at the death, for it seemed to me that such was only to be expected. The only deaths that caused trauma were those of animals caused by human cruelty; witness the copious tears shed reading *Black Beauty*. However, being a big cry-baby Piscean, I also cried a great deal over Life's constant injustices to myself, and true, I did weep copiously at the death of Nancy in *Oliver Twist*. Come to think of it, I have even been known to blubber in a Jeanette McDonald and Nelson Eddy movie, so a great deal of my early life was spent wallowing in salty wetness.

Despite these admissions, I maintain that my nature is, essentially, sanguine and much of that misery is entirely circumstantial and justified. Indeed, you should see how quickly I cheer up with a shift in the situation. How else would I have survived the slings and arrows dealt so continuously and have rebounded so robustly? Yet I did get cancer, didn't I? And I think that it's possibly the stress of that emotional spectrum, which extends the Bell Curve by several grades combined with a more than usually stressful life.[3] For me, highs and lows enter an extremity that has prompted an informal Bipolar II diagnosis. My GP calls this condition *The Artists Disorder*, which explains the complex range of sensibilities many artists share and certainly applies to me.

Until I took myself in hand during my early thirties I would frequently be overwhelmed by sheer emotion, whether it be ecstatic or desolation. During a depressed adolescence, trapped in an impossible domestic situation, *Death* achieved the comforting, almost desirable allure that was eluded only by virtue of an indestructible constitution. Since then, *Death* has been in perennial contemplation, inducing an almost mediaeval sentience of its omnipresence.[4] As a mature student I included *Dying and Bereavement* in my undergraduate Psychology major, filling my journal with Gary Larson cartoons,[5] and I do love the writer, Terry Pratchett's, humorous spin on Death, whose philosophical existentialism almost matches my own.[6]

As a baby-boomer often accused of thinking too much, coupled with acute awareness of the human population's

---

3. Recent research has shown many women attribute their breast cancer to such conditions, rather than accept responsibility for lifestyle choices such as smoking. Whilst I ostensibly accept the figures, I query the conclusions drawn from them, countering that people under stress are more likely to self-medicate with substances such as nicotine.

4. A much more common experience for ancient peoples, Death was always twinned with Life in symbology.

5. Larson has a penchant for cartoons featuring Death with a very ironic twist.

6. In Pratchett's *DiscWorld* series, Death is a long-suffering character with a deep sense of irony, and there is also a character called Death of Rats. In one book, Death gets sick of his job and decides to retire – it's very funny.

rapid escalation, this elicited the convictions that if one could not offer a child a loving, secure home, it was better not to breed, and when Death came knocking one should not argue. I'd intuitively arrived at a sociological observation that the medical maxim of 'Life at any cost' had instigated a death-denying society, encouraging an ultimately futile greed for life. I resolved that when this moment came for me, I would greet Death like a warrior and go without quarrel.

I'd never considered the Big C a possibility. There's no family history, plus I've been such a conscientious avoider of processed and junk food. Expected something more dramatic, like accident or misadventure, but dreamed of a more controlled passing, perhaps winking out like a Zen monk, or singing my death song as the Sioux warriors did. Yet, there I was, actually faced with that very choice, of either 'doing battle with cancer,' a phrase I've long been uncomfortable with, or to let this game follow it's natural course and take lots of nice drugs if there's pain at the end.

I thought, *Here we go, baby! Time to put your money where your mouth has been! Maybe I'll just spend my super, go travelling and wind up on ancestral turf in north-west Scotland at the magical garden of Findhorn,[7] where I'll plant myself with the faeries.*

After that whirlwind of imaginative potentialities, the news from the GP, that the lump was small (10mm), just level two, and not an aggressive type, was an anticlimax. Likewise, with the surgeon, who reckoned it was a done

---

7. Findhorn began with a displaced spiritualist couple who found themselves a home in a caravan park on a stretch of arid, sandy coastline and proceeded to grow a garden with the aid of nature divas that became world famous for its fabulous produce.

deal and I'd be a fool not to go with the plan to remove the lump, along with it's sentinel lymph node,[8] along with some likely radiotherapy. Further reflection determined I was yet to produce my best work in my third career as an author, which had barely begun. Given the prognosis did not include playing King Canute in an arduous war with the inevitable and hanging around for just another cup of tea, I may as well run with it.

So, there I was, seemingly with the best of all possible cancers and an easy out of the mortal choice I'd been gearing up for. We know that nicotine reduces the amount of oxygen carried in the blood, and my blood is going to need all the oxygen it can get. So, if my society was prepared to go to this expense to save my life, I supposed I might as well assist by giving up smoking. I'd never been a heavy smoker, done lots of compensating exercise, and thoroughly enjoyed each one of the daily three to four. Nonetheless, recognising the counterproductive health effects, quitting was an occasional consideration. However, as the antismoking hyperbole grew, smoking had become as much a matter of resistance to this increasing Nanny State invasion of personal preferences as a habit. It seemed to me that it gave many people an accessible target upon which to lay diffuse frustrations. In fact, stopping smoking was simple. I just stopped. Still think I'd like one now and then, but since I'm committed to this bargain I've made with my society, I figure I have to play my part and help this healing along.

It all happened so quickly, just under two weeks from detection to removal. The surgery at Hornsby Hospital

---

8. Have just heard recent research says the removal of the lymph node has been shown to be unnecessary, but ah well, too late for mine.

was a neat overnight stay, the lymph node proved clear, and I'm up for radiotherapy five days per week for four weeks. As far as I'm concerned, I *had* cancer, it went with the lump, and the radiotherapy is to prevent the little bugger from coming back. The one-hour each-way drive to Royal North Shore Hospital for four weeks is tedious, but the two-bus, two-plus hour each way trip would be worse. And all the RNSH Oncology staff are such kind, lovely people. Indeed, they are so inveterately cheerful that I suspect professional development classes at Cheery School.

I've decided that I love nurses.

*Postscript:* I was living in varied temporary situations whilst much of this was occurring, a product of Sydney's housing crisis. My RNSH social worker had arranged for me to stay at Blue Gum Cottage, the hospital's residential accommodation that provides affordable digs for distance patients. Fortunately, I found a home before radiotherapy began. However, that option will not be available to anyone soon, as Blue Gum Cottage has been bought by a private organisation. This is a devastating event for distance patients, most of whom cannot afford commercial rates. So if any readers are seeking a philanthropic venture, I can highly recommend providing RNSH with a replacement patient accommodation.

# Second Opinion Required

*David Howell*

As an Emergency Operations Group Manager, I'd always had an 'open door' policy, which allowed any staff across the Ambulance Service to call by if they had any issues that others in the Service could not assist them with. I was also heavily involved in our peer support and Critical Incident Stress programs, which gave me an advantage over many others.

Staff, although an organisation's greatest resource, are often only seen as a means to an end in many organisations or, by many managers. I was therefore very privileged to have a good rapport with all ambulance staff and I enjoyed meeting them, hearing about their professional and personal lives, and assisting where I could. Ambulance is a caring industry so I worked on the major premise 'that we must take care of our own'.

I was sitting in my office finalising my monthly report when a young paramedic called by to see me. I pushed aside my keyboard in order to give her my full attention; I could see that she was upset. She had already closed the office door. I looked at her as she sat on the well-worn visitor's chair; clearly her normally bright, bubbly personality had an ominous shadow cast across it. She informed me that she had breast cancer, and that she was booked for surgery in a fortnight and would be on sick leave for some weeks. She was extremely worried how all this would impact on her paramedic career as she was still in training and not qualified.

I allayed her fears about her career, because student paramedics moved in and out of their training squads for various reasons, especially sick leave, so it didn't really matter. At hearing this she became teary, as this had been all she'd been really concerned about – her paramedic career. She was worried that she would have to leave. We talked at length about how her training was going and about some jobs and clearly this made her feel a little better and she now had hope – her job was safe!

She then started talking about her cancer and how she had seen a specialist, how everything had happened so quickly and that it had taken her a while to tell her mother. She told me that the surgeon was going to do a full mastectomy. Inwardly, I was churning. Here was a young woman in the prime of her life, in a new career, about to undergo radical breast surgery. I thought of her future and the impact this surgery and therapy would have on her physically and emotionally, how it could potentially affect her self-image, her search for a partner, raising a family and many other aspects of life. I didn't know if she'd had any counselling about the future or if she had even thought about it herself. My mind raced, trying to think of everything, or anything, that might help this vulnerable woman sitting clutching her hands in her lap.

I asked her if she had sought a second opinion. She looked at me blankly, then said that she hadn't because the surgeon had been quite clear that a radical mastectomy was the only treatment. She asked me why I thought of a second opinion. I told her that lumpectomies were sometimes performed instead of radical mastectomies. She was unaware of this, and had never even heard of the term 'lumpectomies'. I explained what the procedures were and strongly suggested that she try and get a second or third opinion on her treatment options, explaining that she was a young woman and she needed to be fully informed of all the issues involved, the prognosis, the treatment options and any after effects.

Whether any of these had been discussed with her I didn't know and she didn't appear to have taken them in, if they had been mentioned. I offered to make some inquiries to see if I could find out names of specialists through some of my medical contacts, but she was happy to follow up this herself.

When she stood to leave I could see that physically she didn't look as vulnerable as she had when she'd entered. Over the next few hours, in between emergency cases, she managed to arrange an appointment with another specialist.

Two days later, the young paramedic informed me that she had seen her new specialist and that she was booked for surgery; the new specialist had decided that a lumpectomy was the preferred treatment option in her case.

The young paramedic recovered well, returned to work and completed her training, becoming a qualified ambulance paramedic. She sent me a thank you card, which I cherished. We often saw each other at emergency scenes or when I visited my ambulance stations and occasionally I would ask how she was going but mostly it was work as usual. I knew by her work ethic and complimentary letters from patients that she was a credit to her profession.

I occasionally think of this young paramedic, helping others in their emergencies or family crises, who needed help herself. We are not alone; there is always someone we can get information or assistance from.

Remember to be fully informed of all aspects of your cancer, the prognosis, the treatment, the after-effects, any support agencies, groups or counselling available.

If you don't know or understand something, ASK!

# The Weight of Breasts

*Vicki Thornton*
*for R*

the words will not be uttered
swells her tongue with fear
leaving a bitter taste

she has parts of herself
methodically removed
*it's not that bad*
she says

standing side on
before a mirror
she runs a hand over her
newly carved lines

*but it makes my arse look big*
she mutters
remembering
the weight of breasts

# Glossary

*The following is by no means intended to offer exhaustive definitions, but are merely quick explanations to facilitate your reading and understanding.*

**Adenocarcinoma** – a cancer that originates in the glandular tissue.

**Adjuvant Therapy** – treatment given in addition to main treatment.

*Anastrozole (also Arimidex)* – a medication used to treat women with breast cancer who have experienced menopause.

**Aspirate** – the removal of fluid and cells through a needle.

**Biopsy** – a medical test in which cells or tissues are taken for examination.

**Cannula** – a tube inserted into the body, usually to deliver fluid or gather data.

**Carcinoma** – the most common type of cancer that occurs in humans. Carcinomas invade tissues and organs and may spread to lymph nodes and elsewhere.

**'Chemo Brain'** – a term used to describe memory, thinking problems and general fogginess, that can occur following cancer treatment.

**Chemotherapy** – a cancer treatment that involves one or more types of drugs that interfere with fast-growing cells, and which is usually given via IV infusion, or can be given orally or infused directly into the limb or liver.

*Dexamethasone* – a drug, which acts as an anti-inflammatory and immuno-suppressant.

*Dolasetron* – a medication used to treat nausea and vomiting following chemotherapy.

**Ductal Carcinoma** – a tumour in the duct.

*Endone* – a medicine used to relieve moderate to severe pain.

**Faith** – believe in yourself and those around you.

*Fosamax* – a drug used in the treatment of Osteoporosis.

**Haematoma** – a swelling which contains blood.

**Hope** – something to hold onto, no matter what.

**Invasive Ductal Carcinoma** – involves an invasive, malignant propagation of cells in breast tissue.

*Kytril* – a medication used to treat nausea and vomiting following chemotherapy.

**Lumpectomy** – a surgical procedure in which a lump is removed from a person's breast.

**Lymphodema** – a condition involving localised fluid retention or tissue swelling caused by a compromised lymphatic system.

**Mammogram** – the use of low-energy X-rays to examine the human breast.

**Mastectomy** – the removal of one or both breasts, in part or in full.

**Metastasise** – to spread through the body.

**Nuclear Medicine** – a branch of medicine, which involves the use of radioactive isotopes in the diagnosis and treatment of cancer.

**Oncology** – a branch of medicine, which deals with cancer.

**Oncologist** – a doctor who deals with cancer

*Ondansetron* – a medication used to treat nausea and vomiting following chemotherapy.

**Osteoporosis** – a disease of the bones that leads to an increased chance in fractures.

*Paclitaxel* – a drug given to treat breast cancer, (as well as ovarian and non-small cell lung cancer).

**Pathology** – the study and diagnosis of disease.

**Pericarditis** – an inflammation of the fibrous sac which surrounds the heart (the pericardium). Often, chest pain is present.

*Phenergan* – a drug given for anticholinergic , antiemetic (against nausea and vomiting), and anti-motion purposes. It also has sedative effects.

**Prophylaxis** – a procedure to prevent, rather than treat or cure, a disease.

**Radical Mastectomy** – the removal of one or both breasts, the underlying chest muscle and lymph nodes.

**Radiotherapy** – the use of ionising radiation to kill cancer cells.

**Remember** – all those who have fought breast cancer.

**Stage 1, 2, 3, 4 Cancer** – a classification for the amount the cancer has spread, with 4 having the most progression.

*Tamoxifen* – a medication used in the treatment of breast cancer, which is oestrogen-dependent.

*Valium* – a sedative.

# Early Detection is Vital

*This fact sheet was reproduced with the permission of
Cancer Council Australia. It can be found on the web at:
www.cancer.org.au*

## Early detection of breast cancer

The chance of a woman developing breast cancer up to age
85 is 1 in 9. Over 12,000 women are diagnosed each year in
Australia. When breast cancer is detected early, women have
a much greater chance of being treated successfully and for
most women the cancer will not come back after treatment.

Screening mammograms are currently the best method
available for detecting breast cancer early. Mammograms
may find a breast cancer which is too small to feel.

## What is a screening mammogram?

Mammograms are low dose x-rays of a woman's breasts.
Screening mammograms are performed on women without
any symptoms of breast cancer. They are provided free of
charge from the BreastScreen Australia program. Women
over 50 years of age are advised to have a mammogram
every two years.

## Who should have a regular screening mammogram?

The biggest risk factors for developing breast cancer are
being a woman and getting older. BreastScreen Australia
targets women aged 50 to 69 years as 75 per cent of all breast
cancers occur in women over the age of 50 years.

- Screening mammograms are often less reliable for
  women under 40 years of age. The density of breast
  tissue in younger women often makes it difficult to
  detect cancers on mammograms.

- All women aged 40 to 49 years who have no breast
  symptoms also have free access to the BreastScreen

Australia program should they choose to a have a screening mammogram.

- All women aged 50 to 69 years are encouraged to have a free mammogram every two years through BreastScreen Australia.

- Women aged over 70 years who have no breast symptoms also have free access to the BreastScreen Australia program. They should discuss whether to have a mammogram with their doctor.

## Where can I have a screening mammogram?

BreastScreen is a free nationally accredited screening program. To contact your local BreastScreen service, call 13 20 50 for the cost of a local call.

There are currently over 500 screening locations including mobile screening units covering rural and remote areas across Australia.

## What if I have a family history of breast cancer?

Breast cancer is a common disease in Australian women. By chance some women will have a relative who has had breast cancer, however less than five per cent of all breast cancers are caused by a family history.

If you have a family history of breast cancer and are concerned about your risk speak to your doctor.

## What to look out for

Women of all ages should be familiar with the normal look and feel of their breasts. If you notice any of the following changes please see your doctor immediately:

- A lump, lumpiness or thickening of the breast.

- Changes in the skin of a breast, such as puckering, dimpling or a rash.

- Persistent or unusual breast pain.

- A change in the shape or size of a breast.
- Discharge from a nipple, a nipple rash or a change in its shape.

## What else can I do?

- Maintain a healthy body weight
- Be physically active on most, preferably all days.
- Eat for health – choose a varied diet with plenty of fruit and vegetables.
- Limit your alcohol intake. The more you drink the greater your risk of developing cancer. If you don't drink don't start. If you choose to drink – no more than one standard drink per day.

Remember, if you have any concerns or questions, please contact your doctor.

## Where can I get reliable information?

**Cancer Council Helpline 13 11 20**
Information and support for you and your family for the cost of a local call anywhere in Australia.

**Cancer Council Australia website**
(with links to state and territory Cancer Councils)
www.cancer.org.au

**BreastScreen Australia 13 20 50**
www.breastscreen.info.au

**National Breast and Ovarian Cancer Centre**
www.nbocc.org.au

*Cancer Council Australia acknowledges the contribution of BreastScreen WA in developing this fact sheet.*

A percentage of profits from this book will be donated
to BreaCan and WHOW.

BreaCan is an information and support service for
people (and their families and friends) affected by a
gynaecological cancer or breast cancer.
It is a statewide service available to people
throughout Victoria.
www.breacan.org.au


WHOW (Women Helping Other Women)
helps provide improved breast cancer services in
areas of need such as Bali.
www.whow.com.au

www.ingramcontent.com/pod-product-compliance
Lightning Source LLC
Chambersburg PA
CBHW022137020426
42334CB00015B/927